DESSERT KETO COOKBOOK 2021

60 sweet recipes,
tasty and low-calorie recipes
to lose weight in a healthy and fast
way with the ketogenic diet

Dr. Grace Roberts Health

TABLE OF CONTENT

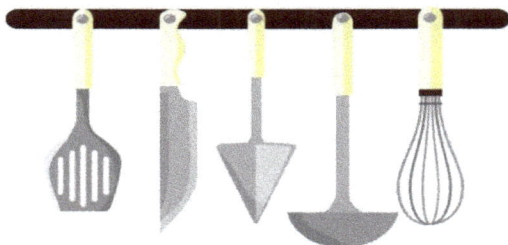

CHERRY CAKE AND COCOA CREAM

Low-carb desserts are increasingly sought after, because finally today we are increasingly aware that our health depends on our diet and even when we are well it is essential to eat healthy.
If you want a healthy and light dessert, but also greedy and beautiful as a presentation, get ready to make this cake.
This soft dessert is low-carb that is low in carbohydrates, paleo, low glycemic content, gluten and lactose free, therefore satisfies everyone's needs since today there are more and more people suffering from intolerances and discovering food allergies.
The peculiarity of this cake lies in the fact that it is created thanks to the filling mold, this mold has a groove on the base, which allows, once the cake has been turned upside down, to fill it by inserting the filling you prefer, chocolate, cream or jam, into a hollow.

Times:
Preparation 50 min
Cooking 20 min
Total 70 min

For 8 people

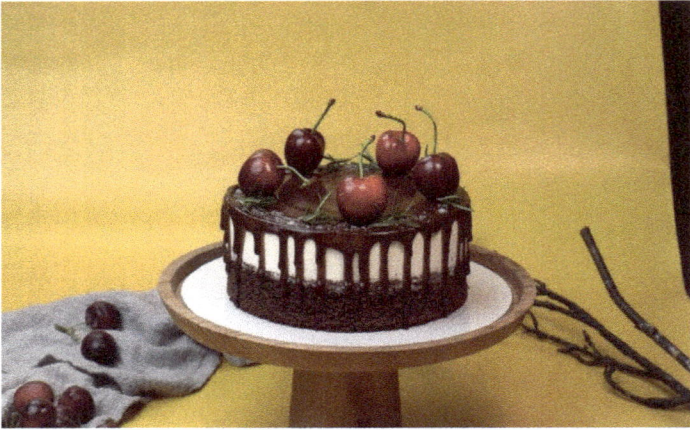

For 1 person:

Nutritional values

Calories 320

Carbohydrates 6.27 gr

Ratio 2.86 gr

Fats 16 gr

Protein 8.49 gr

MATERIALS

Electric whips

1 mold for filling of 26 cm

Mixer or food processor

1 bowl

INGREDIENTS

4 medium eggs

50 grams of almonds

60 gr dried-rasped or rapé grated coconut

15 grams of fine coconut flour

50 grams of coconut sugar

1 teaspoon of cinnamon

80 grams of coconut oil or soft ghee butter

500 gr of fresh cherries

sliced almonds to taste

10 gr of baking powder or cream of tartar

500 gr of cocoa custard

For the syrup:

a teacup of warm water with

1 teaspoon of cocoa e

1 large teaspoon of honey

optional 1 tablespoon of liqueur such as rum,

Grand Marnier or Cherry

Marjoram or thyme for the garnish

INSTRUCTIONS

First, grease the filling mold and flour it with fine coconut flour, turn on the convection oven at 170 degrees for 10 minutes. With a mixer or a food processor, chop and mix well the almonds with the rapé coconut and coconut flour, then add all the other ingredients, except for the yeast and mix making sure to mix well, now you can also add the yeast. , add it to the rest of the ingredients and pour everything into the 26 cm filling mold, place in a ventilated oven at 170 ° degrees for about 20 minutes, in the meantime wash and dry the cherries thoroughly and set them aside in a bowl.

Then prepare the cocoa custard, about 500 gr.

Remove the cake from the oven only after doing the toothpick test * to see if it is cooked, let it cool and then remove it gently from the mold,

now in a pan lightly toast the sliced almonds and put them on one side, you will only need them at the end.

Prepare the syrup by mixing hot water with cocoa and honey, taste and, if necessary, adjust according to your taste.

When the cake has cooled, you will place it on a nice serving dish or a cake stand, sprinkle the syrup especially on the edges of the tart and only a little in the center, pour the cream into the center of the cake, level everything and decorate with imagination, with cherries and sliced almonds.

* Toothpick test:

Pierce the cake / dessert with a toothpick if it comes out and nothing sticks, it means that it is cooked.

Note

We will keep the cake with cocoa cream and cherries in the fridge and we will keep it at room temperature for about 15-20 minutes before serving. You can replace cherries with strawberries, blackberries, figs or even better with fresh raspberries.

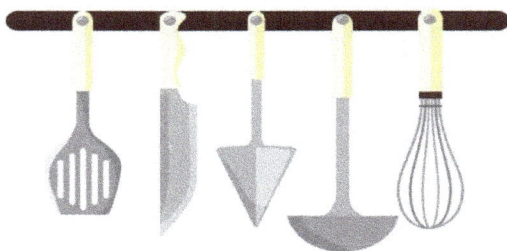

TIRAMISU'

Tiramisu is a famous Italian dessert and certainly one of the tastiest ever. This reinterpretation of the original recipe does not include the use of sugar or the classic ladyfingers, but rather low-carb ladyfingers and sugar substitutes, allowing you to significantly lower the amount of carbohydrates and calories without compromising the taste. As an alternative to lady finger you can use low-carb pavesini, for a slightly more delicate taste.

Times:

Preparation 30 min

Total 30 min

For 6 people

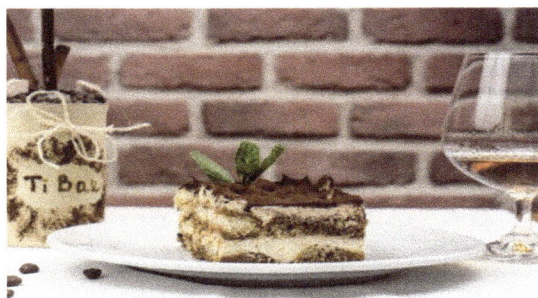

For 1 person:

Nutritional values

Calories 340

Net carbohydrates 5 gr

Fiber 5 gr

Protein 9 gr

Fat 38 gr

MATERIALS

Rectangular ceramic or disposable bowl

Electric or hand whips

Small saucepan

INGREDIENTS

24 low carb ladyfingers

4 Organic eggs (very fresh)

75 gr Erythritol

30 ml Water

20 drops Vanilla liquid Stevia

350 gr Mascarpone

Cocoa powder to taste

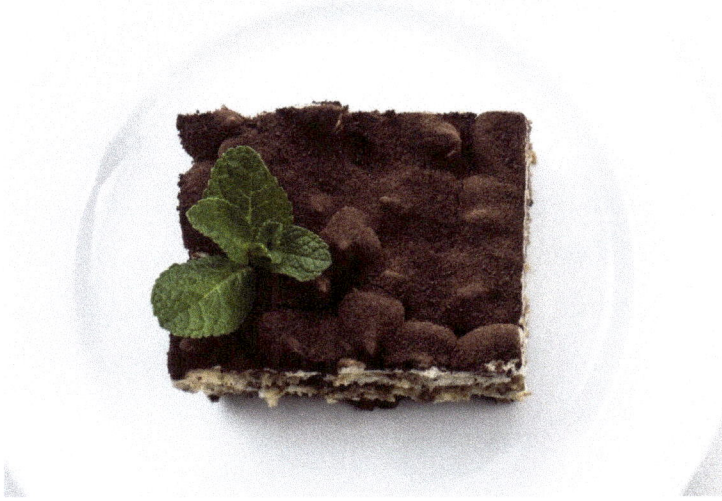

INSTRUCTIONS

First prepare some coffee, about 3/4 cups according to your tastes, add some liqueur to the coffee (optional) with 10 g of erythritol and a few drops of liquid stevia, now put it on one side and leaveat it to cool. Now prepare some syrup by heating 30 ml of water with 65 g of erythritol in a saucepan, until it boils and the erythritol has dissolved completely. This operation of adding the syrup to the eggs will serve to pasteurize them and be quiet, even if with fresh and organic eggs you will certainly have no problem. In the meantime, separate the egg whites from the yolks, and when the syrup has reached the boil, whisk the egg whites, adding half the syrup little by little. Once the egg whites have been whipped, bring the other half of the syrup to the boil and then whip the yolks as well, adding the syrup little by little, now add the mascarpone to the yolks little by little with 15/20 drops of liquid stevia. When the mixture is homogeneous, slowly add the previously whipped egg whites. To assemble the tiramisu, start with a light layer of cream on the bottom in a rectangular or disposable aluminum bowl. Soak the ladyfingers well in the coffee and form a base with the biscuits, adding a generous layer of cream on top, repeat the process with layers of ladyfingers and cream, finish with a layer of cream with a generous sprinkling of bitter cocoa on top. The number of layers of ladyfingers and cream ranges from a minimum of 3 at will. Let the tiramisu rest in the refrigerator for at least 4 hours, preferably 8 hours for a better result.

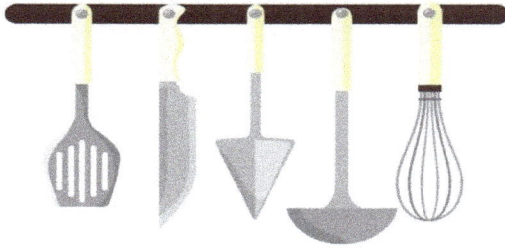

KETO NUTELLA

Getting close to the flavor of the original Nutella recipe is really difficult, but in this recipe the healthy / flavor compromise has been definitely reached, Keto Nutella is super greedy, you will be happily surprised.

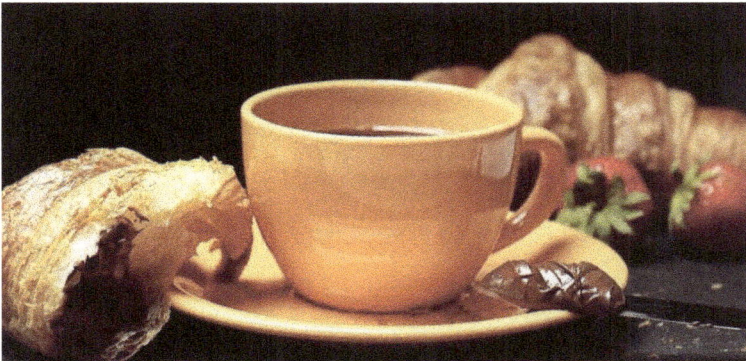

Times:

Preparation 20 min

Cooking 11 minutes

Total 31 min

For 2 jars

For 1 jar:

Nutritional values

Calories 140

Net carbohydrates 4 gr

Fiber 8 gr

Protein 7 gr

Fat 6 gr

MATERIALS

2 glass jars

Mixer

1 small saucepan

INGREDIENTS

1 cup of walnuts (130 g)

1 cup of shelled hazelnuts (150 g)

1/2 cup almonds (75 g)

1 85-90% dark chocolate bar (100 gr)

1 tablespoon of coconut oil (15 g)

2 tablespoons of powdered Erythritol (20 g)

(sweetener, optional)

1 tablespoon of 100% pure cocoa powder (5 g)

vanilla to taste

INSTRUCTIONS

Put the hazelnuts, almonds and walnuts in the oven for 9-11 minutes at 180 ° degrees, when they are well toasted let them cool, then melt the dark chocolate in a microwave or in a bain-marie.

Blend the hazelnuts, almonds and walnuts and add the melted chocolate, cocoa powder, coconut oil, erythritol, vanilla extract, all in the blender and blend again.

When you reach the right density pour it into glass jars, which can be stored for a long time, by doing this, cap them and put them back in hot water for 45 minutes, so they will be vacuum-packed, to be consumed when you prefer.

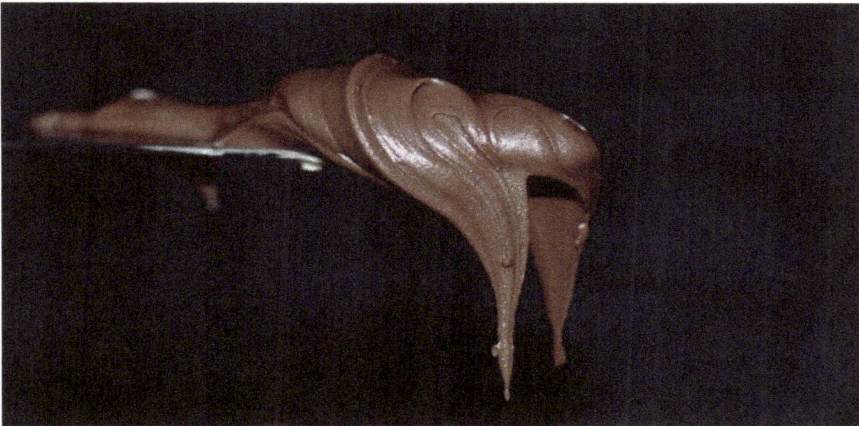

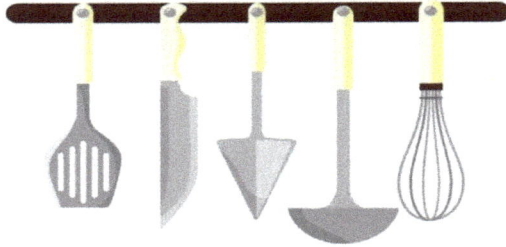

COCONUT CREPES

Coconut crepes are very easy to make and absolutely delicious, in this case albeit to be eaten within a ketogenic regime comparable in taste to the original recipe.

Times:

Preparation 10 min

Cooking 3 min

Total 13 min

For 4 people

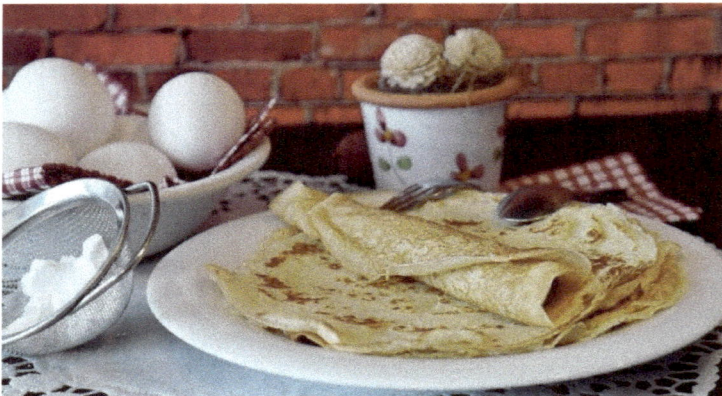

For 1 crepe:

Nutritional values

Calories 183

Net carbohydrates 12 gr

Sugars 5 gr

Fiber 4 gr

Protein 9 gr

Fat 3 gr

MATERIALS

Non-stick pan or specific for crepes

Electric or hand whips

1 bowl

INGREDIENTS

Egg white 200 ml

Whey natural chocolate protein 10 gr

30 gr Chopped hazelnuts

10 gr Chopped coconut

10 gr Bitter cocoa

Sweetener to taste

INSTRUCTIONS

Put the whey, egg whites and sweetener in a bowl and mix very slowly, making sure to mix the mixture well so as not to have lumps.

The mixture obtained, pour it into a non-stick pan, or specific for crepes, cook the dough for a few seconds until it is golden.

Take the crepe obtained and sprinkle it with a part of chopped hazelnuts and chopped coconut, close it in the shape of a fan and sprinkle over the coconut and the remaining hazelnuts and sprinkle with bitter cocoa.

Serve it hot / lukewarm.

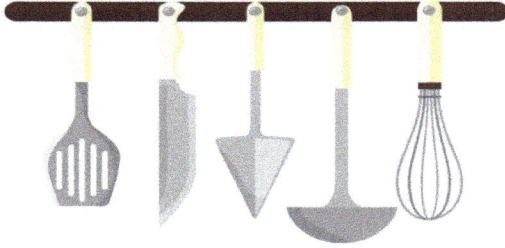

KETO CUSTARD CREAM

This recipe is also perfect for anyone who wants to maintain a healthy diet.

Low-carb and in ketogenic version it is quick and easy to prepare, excellent for filling sweets, cakes, biscuits or you can eat it alone with a spoon.

Times:

Preparation 10 min

Cooking 15 min

Total 25 min

For 6 people (500 gr)

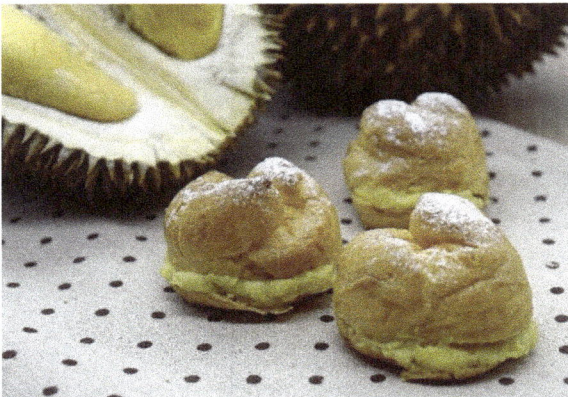

P.for 1 portion:

Nutritional values

Calories 144

Total carbohydrates 16 gr

Protein 3.99 gr

Fat 4 gr

MATERIALS

Electric whips

1 saucepan

1 bowl

INGREDIENTS

6 yolks

100 gr Tagatesse or Erythritol (sweetener powder)

100 ml Almond milk or unsweetened coconut milk

100 gr Soft butter

A envelope of vanillin

INSTRUCTIONS

Put the egg yolks and the sweetener in a thick-bottomed, non-stick pan and mix well, well, eliminating any lumps.

Add the almond milk (make sure it does not contain added sugar) and finally the vanillin.

Cook over low heat making sure it does not burn or stick to the bottom.

Cook for a few minutes, until you have obtained a smooth and homogeneous creamy consistency, then remove the pot from the heat and let it cool.

When the mixture is well cooled, add the butter and whisk everything with an electric blender, at medium speed.

This recipe is very easy to make and can be used to dress desserts, garnish or excellent to eat by the spoon.

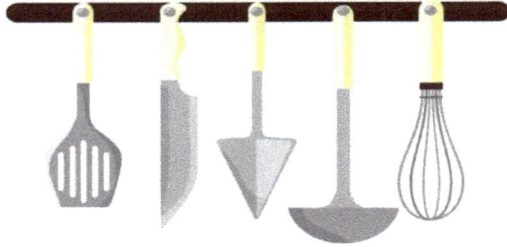

CHOCOLATE MUFFIN

Muffins are perfect for any occasion, in this recipe they are chocolate, particularly suitable for breakfast, gluten-free, low-carb and ketogenic.

Times:

Preparation 15 min

Cooking 40 min

Total 55 min

For 12 muffins

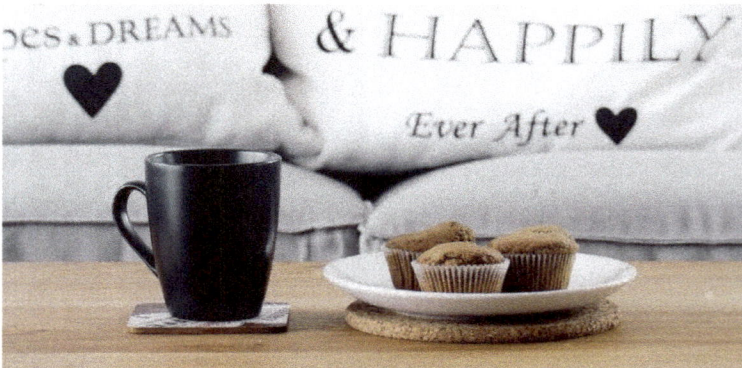

For 1 muffin:

Nutritional values

Calories 340

Net carbohydrates 4.5 / 100 gr

Fibers 3.8 / 100 gr

Protein 5.6 gr

Fat 3.8 gr

Polyols 18/100 gr

MATERIALS

Electric whips

Sieve

Small saucepan

2 Bowls

12 muffin cups

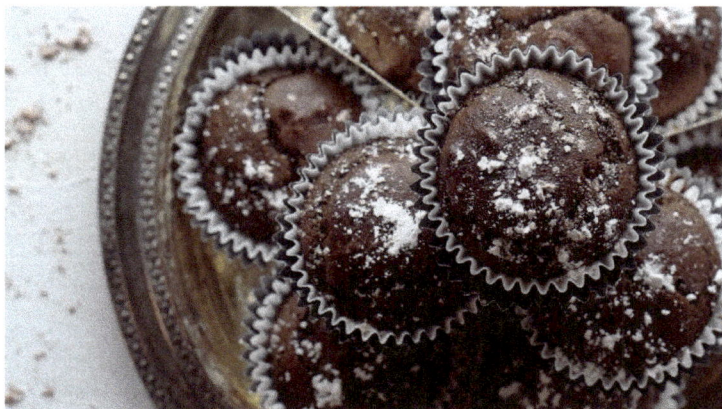

INGREDIENTS

50 g Almond Flour

50 g Coconut Flour

200 ml Cream

3 eggs

50 g Butter (melted)

20 g Cocoa powder

150 g Erythritol

10 drops liquid stevia with chocolate

1/2 tsp Yeast

1 pinch Salt

INSTRUCTIONS

In a bowl add the cream, eggs, soft / melted butter, erythritol and liquid stevia, mix with an electric whisk at medium speed, until the mixture becomes homogeneous, at the same time in another bowl sift the coconut flour, almonds and cocoa and add the yeast and a pinch of salt.

Separate the mixture and pour it into about 12 medium-sized muffin cups.

Bake in the oven at 180 degrees for 35-40 minutes.

Serve them lukewarm.

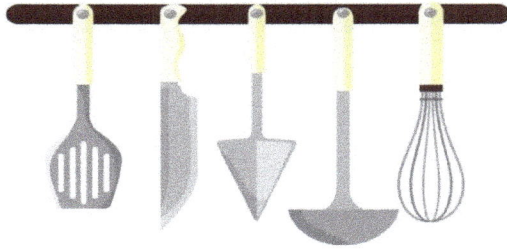

TASTY CHOCOLATE CAKE

The gluttonous chocolate cake is a cake made with almond flour with a very rich taste, in this recipe the use of traditional sugar is not foreseen, thus making it low-carb and perfectly compatible with the ketogenic diet, while maintaining a truly flavor greedy, like its name.

Times:

Preparation 30 min

Cooking 30 min

Total 60 min

For 10 people

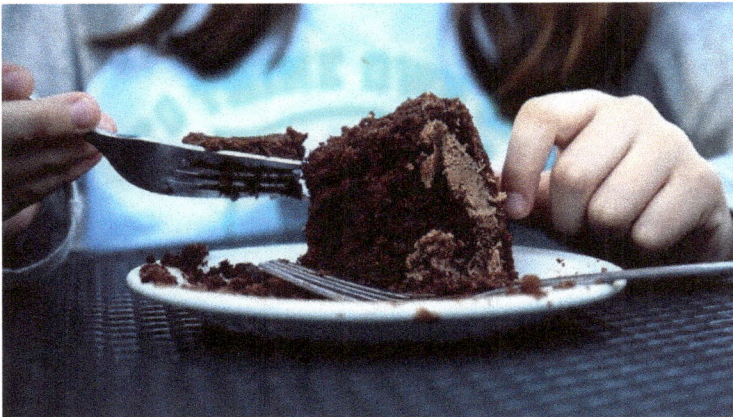

For 1 slice:

Nutritional values

Calories 324

Net carbohydrates 6/25 gr

Total 13 gr

Fiber 7 gr

Polyols 15 gr

Protein 9.7 / 100 gr

Fats 29.3 / 166 gr

MATERIALS

Electric or hand whips

Cake pan diameter 26/28 cm

Small saucepan

2 Bowls

INGREDIENTS

For the chocolate

150 g Cocoa paste

50 g Erythritol powder

10 drops liquid stevia with chocolate

For the cake

180 g Almond flour

125 g Erythritol

200 g Butter

5 Eggs

15 drops Vanilla liquid Stevia

The zest of an orange

INSTRUCTIONS

Melt the cocoa mass with the butter in a microwave or double boiler. Add the erythritol and the liquid stevia, and mix until well incorporated, making sure that there are no lumps, set the chocolate aside and let it cool. Separate the egg whites from the yolks and whisk the egg whites until stiff, beat the yolks with the erythritol until a homogeneous and foamy mixture is formed. Now add the chocolate to the beaten egg whites and mix until well incorporated. Now add the almond flour (preferably sifted) and mix until you get a homogeneous mixture. Now incorporate the egg whites a little at a time. Place the mixture in a pan and cook in a static oven for about 30 minutes at 180 degrees.

After letting the cake cool, sprinkle with powdered erythritol (Optional).

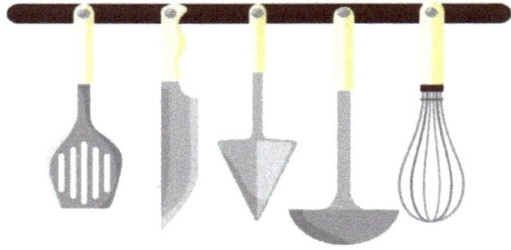

CREAMY CAKE CREAM AND CHOCOLATE

This recipe is quite traditional in taste, not too quick to make, but super rich in flavor while respecting the ketogenic diet regime, it remains a cake suitable for all palates and healthy.

Times:

Preparation 45 min

Cooking 25 min

Total 70 min

For 12 people

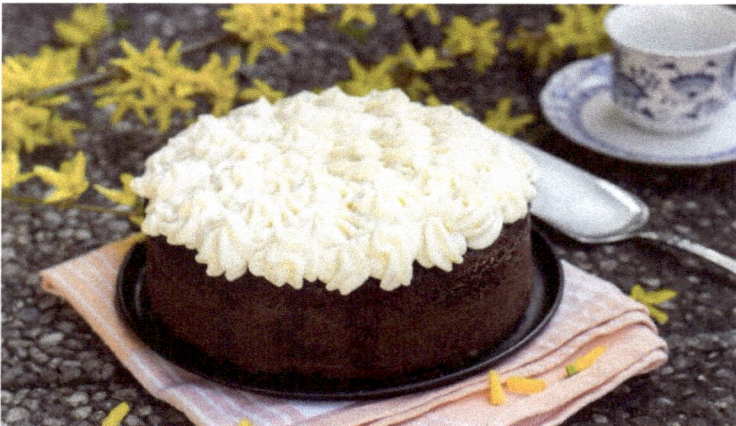

For 1 slice:

Nutritional values

Calories 290

Net carbohydrates 5.8 / 25 gr

Total 11.1 gr

Fiber 5.4 gr

Polyols 18 gr

Protein 6.6 / 100 gr

Fats 25.5 / 166 gr

MATERIALS

Electric whips

Oven dish 24/26 cm

Small saucepan

Bowl or graduated glass

INGREDIENTS

For the base

4 eggs

200 ml Water

80 gr Almond flour

50 gr Coconut flour

15 gr Cocoa powder

50 gr Erythritol

80 ml Almond milk (unsweetened)

1 pinch Salt

1/2 tsp Baking soda (optional)

For the cream layer

30 gr Cream

15 drops Vanilla Stevia

For the chocolate layer

20 ml Cream

100 gr Cocoa paste

80 gr Erythritol powder

10 stevia chocolate drops

50 gr Butter

INSTRUCTIONS

The base

Whip the eggs until the mixture is light and frothy, add the water and mix the mixture, then add the almond flour, coconut, erythritol, cocoa and baking soda and continue stirring. Pour everything into a greased, oiled or parchment paper pan and bake at 180 degrees for about 30 minutes, once ready and passed the toothpick test, let the base cool down well. Spread the almond milk on the cooled base, let it absorb and put it in the fridge.

The cream layer

In a container put 300 ml cream and the vanilla stevia, whip until you get a creamy mixture, add the whipped cream over the base and refrigerate, in the meantime prepare the chocolate layer.

The final layer of chocolate

In a saucepan, boil 200 ml of cream, meanwhile in a container put the cocoa mass, erythritol, stevia with chocolate and butter, add the hot cream and melt everything until you obtain a chocolate ganache, always mixing well, then let it cool for at least 10 minutes in the refrigerator. Spread the chocolate layer over the cream layer trying to cover the cake evenly.

Put the cake in the refrigerator for at least 4 hours before eating it. If you have time, leave it in the fridge overnight and serve it the next day, so it will be perfect.

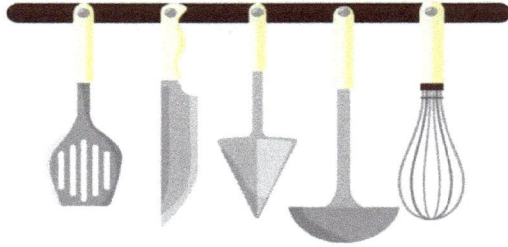

COOKIES WITH CHOCOLATE CHIPS

This is the recipe for a good mood, baking chocolate chip cookies in the Keto version will gratify you at any time of your day.

The flavor is super rich and enhanced by the crunchiness.

Times:

Preparation 15 min

Cooking 12 min

Total 27 min

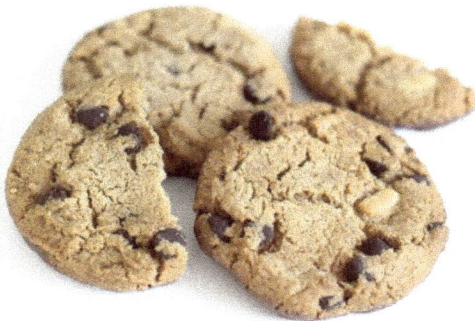

For 2 biscuits:

Nutritional values

Calories 347

Fat 0.6 gr

Fiber 4.4 gr

Sugars 1.3 gr

Polyols 18 gr

Net Carbohydrates 1.7 gr

Protein 8.5 gr

MATERIALS

Baking bowl or parchment paper

Mixer or food processor

INGREDIENTS

200 gr Almond flour

100 gr Granulated Erythritol

5 drops vanilla stevia

1 egg

1 pinch of salt

20 gr Extra dark chocolate chips

INSTRUCTIONS

Preheat the oven to 180 degrees for 10 minutes and in the meantime create an almond paste by chopping the almond flour for 2-3 minutes. The mixture should have a fluid and creamy consistency, add the almond paste with the rest of the ingredients, leave only one part of the chocolate chips.

Have fun giving various shapes to your biscuits, the round one is certainly the simplest, finally add the chocolate chips on top of the mixture, crushing them a little and bake for about 10/12 minutes.

Remove from the oven and serve lukewarm.

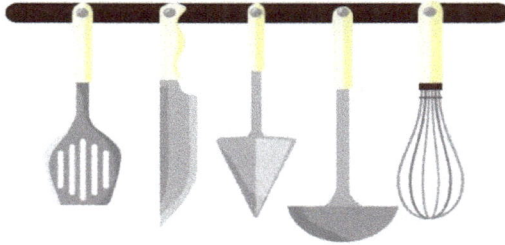

COFFEE BI-DONUT

This is the recipe for the simplest and best known dessert to make, here revisited in a keto version, low-carb, gluten-free, in 2 colors enhanced by the taste of coffee. Soft and particularly digestible suitable for breakfast, snack and all the useful moments for a snack.

Times:

Preparation 25 min

Cooking 40 min

Total 65 min

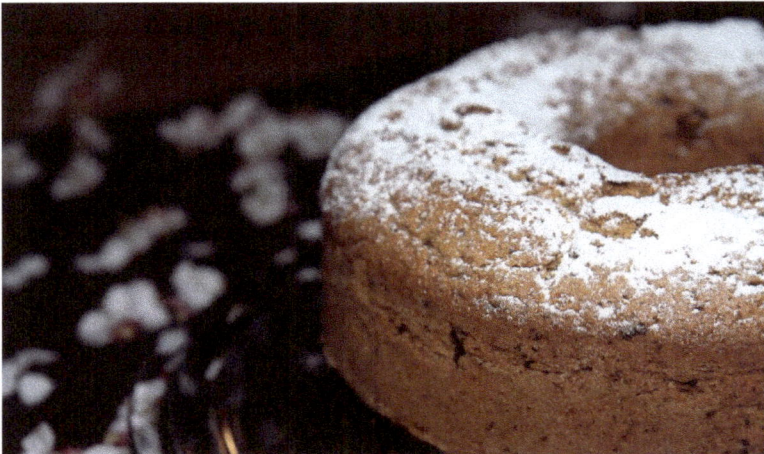

For 10 people

For 1 slice:

Nutritional values

Calories 208

Net carbohydrates 3.2 / 25 gr

Total 5.6 gr

Fiber 2.5 gr

Polyols 15 gr

Protein 5.1 / 100gr

Fats 19.2 / 166 gr

MATERIALS

Electric whips

Oven dish 24/26 cm

2 Bowls

INGREDIENTS

50 gr Almond Flour

50 gr Coconut Flour

150 gr Erythritol

5 Eggs

200 ml Cream

80 gr Butter (melted)

2 cups of espresso

5 gr Cocoa

1 tsp Yeast

1 pinch Salt

INSTRUCTIONS

In a bowl add coconut flour and almond flour (sifted), plus erythritol, baking powder and a pinch of salt, mix well to mix all the ingredients avoiding lumps.

Now add the eggs, cream and melted butter, mix everything until you get a homogeneous mixture.

In a second bowl add 1/3 of the mixture, to this add the 2 cups of espresso and cocoa and continue mixing everything.

Separately add the 2 compounds, the dark and the light one, in a donut mold, (optional) add some sugar-free chocolate chips.

Bake in the oven at 180 degrees for about 40 minutes.

Serve lukewarm.

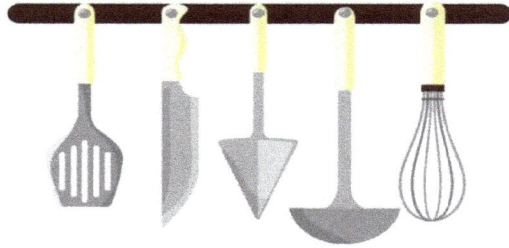

CHOCOLATE ICE CREAM

This recipe is simple, light and fresh for all times: of the day. The basis of the recipe is the same, it can be done in many different tastes.

Times:

Preparation 20 min

Ice cream maker 25 min

Total 45 min

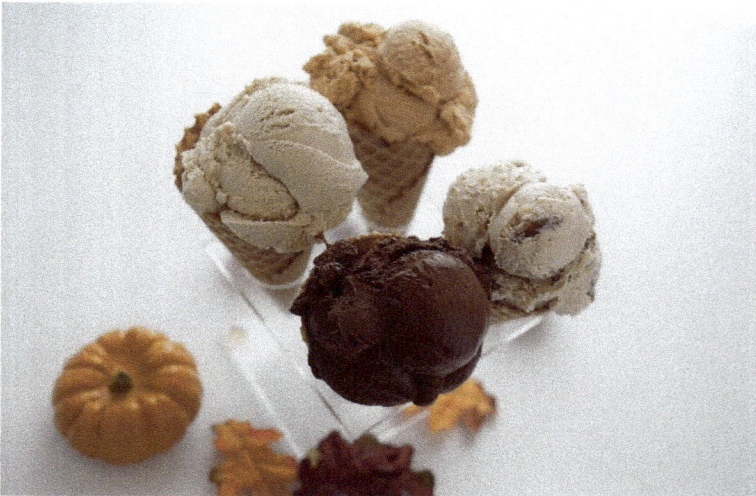

For 10 people

For 1 person (80 gr):

Nutritional values

Calories 190

Net carbohydrates 3.2 gr

Total 4 gr

Fiber 0.8 gr

Polyols 5 gr

Protein 2.1 gr

Fat 19.5 gr

MATERIALS

Ice cream maker

1 small saucepan

Electric whips

1 Strainer

INGREDIENTS

500 ml Cream

200 ml Milk

60 gr Xylitol

15 gr Cocoa paste

10 gr Cocoa powder

5 stevia chocolate drops

1 gr pure Stevia powder

(or you can replace the stevia

with another 50 g of Xylitol)

1/2 tsp Pure vanilla

INSTRUCTIONS

In a saucepan, put 50 ml milk with xylitol, pure stevia, chocolate stevia drops, cocoa mass and vanilla.

Boil until the ingredients have dissolved completely, stirring occasionally. Strain the chocolate mixture just melted and let it cool. In a separate container, lightly whip the 500 ml of cream to thicken it and gradually add the remaining 150 ml of milk. Add the melted chocolate with the cocoa powder to the freshly whipped mixture, mix with the electric whisk until everything is mixed. Add the final mixture into an ice cream machine and let it work for about 25 minutes, or until the ice cream is solid enough.

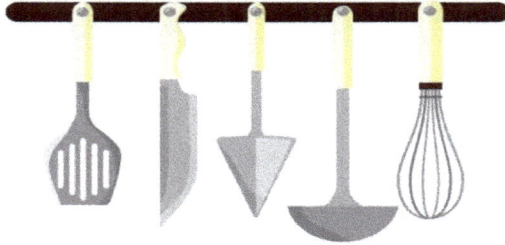

HAZELNUT ICE CREAM

This recipe is simple, light and fresh for all time of the day. The basis of the recipe is the same, it can be made in many different flavors.

Times:

Preparation 20 min

Ice cream maker 20 min

Total 40 min

For 10 people

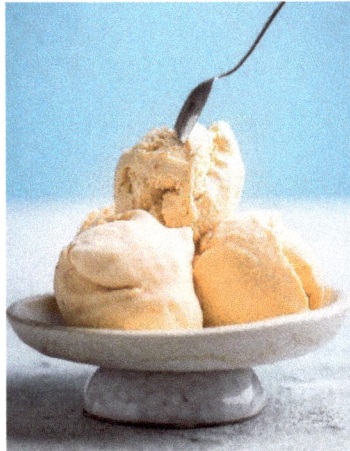

For 1 person (80 gr):

Nutritional values

Calories 247

Net carbohydrates 3.3 gr

Total 4.2 gr

Fiber 1 gr

Polyols 8 gr

Protein 3.11 gr

Fats 25.2 gr

MATERIALS

Ice cream maker

Electric whips

1 small saucepan

1 bowl

1 sieve

INGREDIENTS

500 ml Cream

200 ml Milk

150 gr Hazelnuts

50 gr Xylitol

1 gr pure Stevia powder

(or replace with another

50 gr of Xylitol)

1/2 tsp Pure vanilla

INSTRUCTIONS

In a saucepan put 50 ml milk with xylitol, stevia and vanilla, boil until the ingredients dissolve completely, in a separate container add the cream with the remaining 150 ml of milk. Then add, with the help of a kitchen sieve, the sweeteners previously dissolved in the saucepan, lightly whisk the mixture with an electric mixer until everything is mixed. Chop the hazelnuts until you get a smooth and homogeneous consistency and filter them with a sieve to avoid lumps. To obtain a hazelnut ice cream, add the hazelnut mixture created previously and if you prefer a vanilla ice cream you can skip this point. Finally put the mixture in the ice cream maker and let it go for 15/20 minutes or until the mixture has become solid and creamy. Ready to serve.

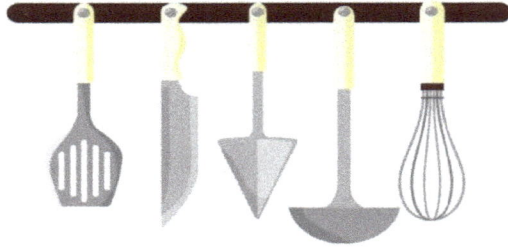

CAKE COFFEE'

This is a recipe that can be prepared in less than 1 hour, particularly suitable as a birthday cake, healthy, low-carb, and perfect as part of a Keto diet.

Times:

Preparation 30 min

Cooking 20 min

Total 50 min

For 12 people

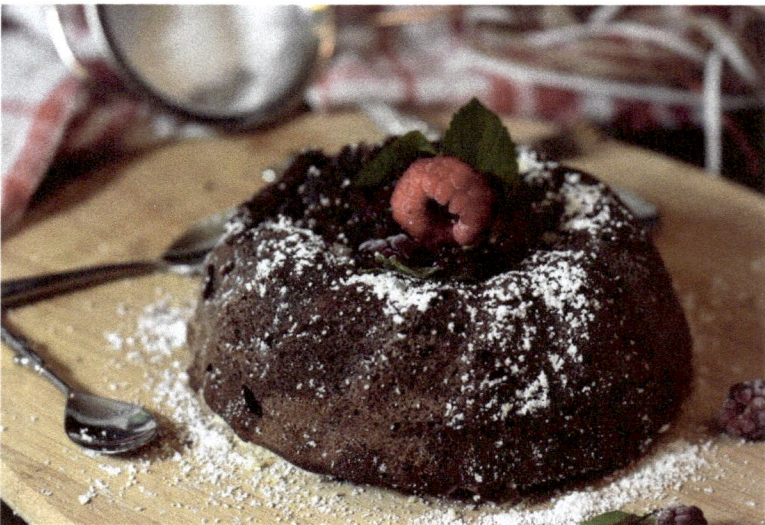

For 1 slice:

Nutritional values

Calories 265

Net carbohydrates 4.5 / 25 gr

Totals. 7.8 gr

Fibers 2.9 gr

Polyols. 18 gr

Proteins. 6.7 / 100 gr

Fat. 30.8 / 166 gr

MATERIALS

Electric whips

2 trays of the same size

1 small saucepan

2 Bowls

INGREDIENTS

For the cake

100 gr Cocoa paste

85 gr Butter

150 gr Erythritol

1 espresso

6 eggs

6 gr Cocoa powder

For the stuffing

400 gr cream

250 gr mascarpone

125 gr Erythritol

1 long espresso

INSTRUCTIONS

For the cake

Preheat the oven to 180 degrees for about 10 minutes and prepare 2 trays of the same size. Melt the butter in a saucepan with the cocoa mass, add an espresso and 50 g of erythritol to the mixture. Separate the yolks and the whites of the 6 eggs. Beat the egg yolks together with 20 grams of erythritol and the cocoa powder, add the melted chocolate at the beginning (making sure it is not yet hot) to the egg whites and cocoa mixture, mix well to mix everything. Beat the egg whites until stiff adding the remaining 80 grams of erythritol, be careful to add them 1/3 at a time, little by little. Incorporate the egg whites into the mixture from bottom to top so as not to dismantle them. Once the egg whites are incorporated, separate the final mixture equally in the 2 trays. Bake for about 20 minutes at 180 degrees.

For the icing

Prepare a double espresso and let it cool in the refrigerator. Beat the cream first until it forms a fairly solid mixture. Add the mascarpone with 125 g of erythritol and beat the mixture until everything is mixed well. Add the cooled coffee and mix the mixture well for the last time. Fill the cake with a generous layer of cream in the middle and cover the rest of the cake with the rest of the cream.

Ready to be served.

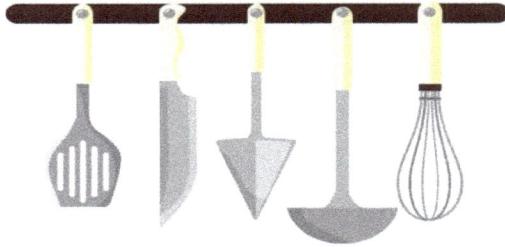

WAFFLE KETO

Ideal for breakfast, as a snack or for a party, this sweet recipe will make you forget you're on a diet. Eat your hot or warm waffles, freshly baked alone or accompanied with raspberries, strawberries and blueberries, they will be a gratification for everyone's palate and as a reward within the ketogenic diet.

Times:

Preparation 6 min

Cooking 15 min

Total 21 min

For 4 people

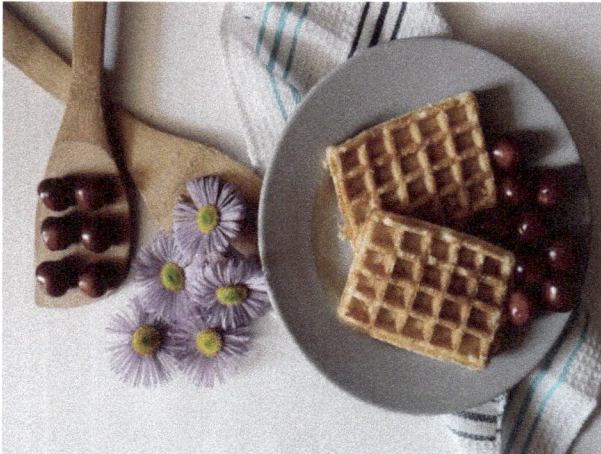

For 1 person:

Nutritional values

Calories 299

Sugars. 1.4 gr

Fats 27.6 gr

Protein 8.9 gr

Carbohydrates 8 gr

MATERIALS

Electric whips

1 Cylindrical container
or large glass

Waffle toaster

INGREDIENTS

360 gr of almond flour

a pinch of salt

4 gr of baking powder

2 tablespoons of erythritol

2 large eggs

200 ml of almond milk

60 gr of extra virgin coconut oil

1 tablespoon of vanilla extract

INSTRUCTIONS

In a cylindrical bowl, beat the eggs until the mixture is firm and foamy, in another bowl pour the almond flour, baking powder and salt, mix and mix all the ingredients together until the mixture is homogeneous. Preheat the plate for a few minutes while the mixture will rest a little, at this point depending on your waffle iron, pour the mixture to cook, on average 5/7 minutes are enough to finish cooking and brown your waffles on both sides.

This delicious recipe is also perfect for making a nice presentation as a family or for a party. Garnish the waffles with strawberries, raspberries, blueberries or Greek yogurt - all healthy and of course, low-carb.

But pay attention to the combinations, because waffles have a lot of carbohydrates so in order not to get out of ketosis you will have to pay close attention to what you will put in combination.

Serve them hot / lukewarm.

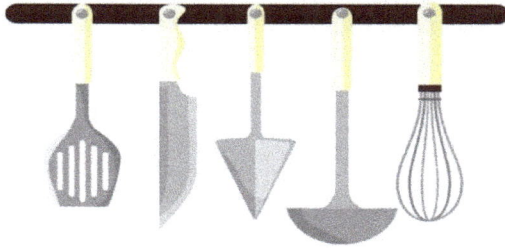

COCONUT SPONGE CAKE

The recipe for this sponge cake is essential for all lovers of sweets, eaten alone or as a base for more elaborate cakes, the result is a very soft base.

It is excellent for breakfast, accompanied by coffee, cappuccino or a delicious cup of tea, or served at the end of a meal, perhaps accompanied by a little whipped cream and fresh blueberries. This low glycemic index recipe will please everyone, from those who follow the keto diet to those who want to eat something healthy but extremely tasty, without flour or gluten.

Times:

Preparation 25 min

Cooking 25 min

Total 50 min

For 12 people

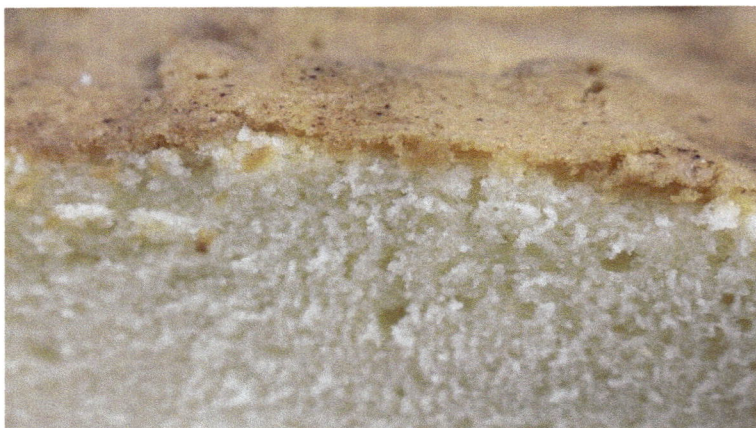

For 1 person:

Nutritional values

178 calories per serving

Sugars 2.6 gr

Fats 16.3 gr

Protein 3.8 gr

MATERIALS

Electric or hand whips

1 Baking terrine 24/25 cm

1 bowl

INGREDIENTS

4 eggs

250 gr coconut flour (or grated coconut)

300 ml of water or other milk replacement drink

(coconut, almond, soy, etc.)

120 grams of Greek yogurt

60 gr of erythritol

1/2 sachet of baking powder

a vanilla bean or unsweetened vanilla flavoring

INSTRUCTIONS

Whisk the egg whites until stiff, add the erythritol to the foam obtained, then add the egg yolks and vanilla, mixing everything vigorously.

Add the milk, coconut flour and Greek yogurt to the mixture, continuing to mix with a spoon to mix all the ingredients.

At this point, turn on the oven and preheat it for 15 minutes at 180 degrees, leaving the mixture to rest in the refrigerator for the same time.

Grease or oil a bowl of about 24/25 cm in diameter, pour all the mixture and cook in the oven, preferably ventilated for 25 minutes.

The coconut sponge cake is the basis for many traditional and famous cakes, because it is soft and tasty, perfect for any filling and filling and above all easy to prepare.

A recipe that must be tried at least once in a lifetime.

One of the biggest surprises you will have when cooking our recipes, once you have started the ketogenic diet, is the possibility of preparing desserts as an alternative to traditional, low glycemic index, gluten free and at the same time very good and beautiful to look at, as in case of the recipe just finished.

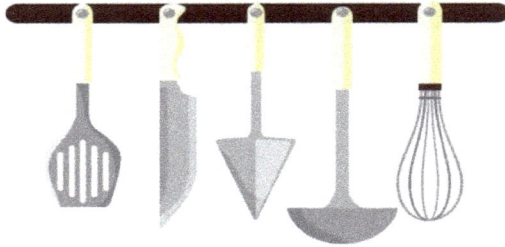

PANCAKE KETO

As you well know, the ketogenic regime helps you to lose weight by not using certain foods such as flour, in favor of many other foods with a high protein index, this recipe is a perfect example.

Times:

Preparation 15 min

Cooking 15 min

Total 30 min

For 4 people

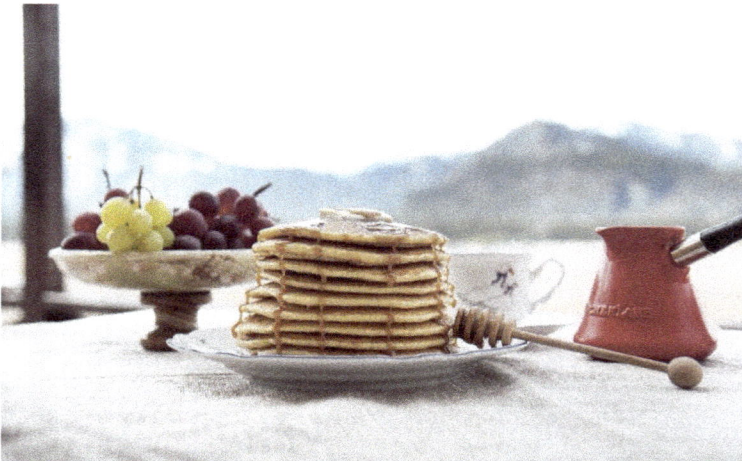

For 1 person:

Nutritional values

Calories 94

Net Carbohydrates 0.3 gr

Fat 8.5 gr

Protein 3.1 gr

MATERIALS

Mixer, electric or hand whisk

1 non-stick pan

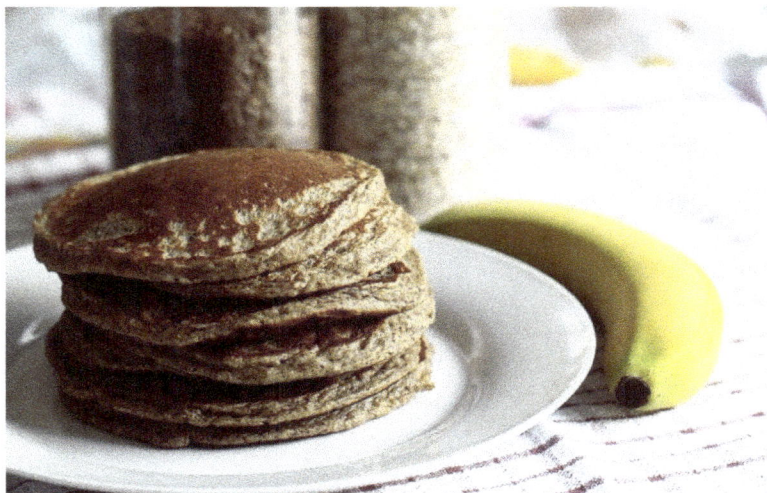

INGREDIENTS

3 medium eggs

1 teaspoon of cinnamon

12 gr of erythriol

4 gr of baking powder

37 gr of finely chopped flax seeds in a blender

30 grams of clarified butter or gaiters

INSTRUCTIONS

Combine all the fat ingredients with the exception of the eggs, mix well with a hand whisk, electric or with the help of a mixer, finally add, when the consistency is creamy, the eggs, continuing to mix until the mixture is uniform.

Let the mixture rest in the fridge for 10 minutes.

Take a non-stick pan and heat it for a few minutes, over medium heat,

once it is hot, pour the mixture to cover the pan with a thin layer and let it brown evenly for about 45 seconds, cook the other side of the pancake for about 30 seconds.

Follow by doing the same thing for how many pancakes you want to bake.

These Pancakes are fluffy and fluffy, perfect for breakfast or served as a dessert.

You can accompany them with Greek yogurt and blueberries or strawberry jam (in the next recipe) or apricots, or simply accompanied by shavings of bitter chocolate.

Serve them lukewarm.

Note:

Those who follow the ketogenic diet will find themselves from time to time wanting to satisfy the desire for sweet.

This keto pancake recipe is pretty simple and the result is surprisingly good.

To make the recipe precious there are the added value of the Omega 3 content and a very low glycemic index 0.1.

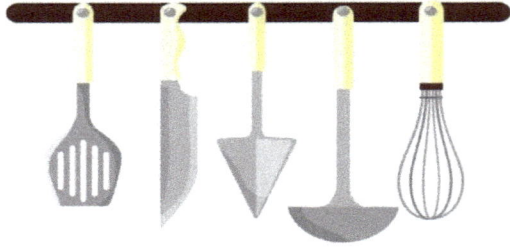

STRAWBERRY JAM

The Chia Seed Strawberry Jam recipe is especially easy to make sugar-free, keto, paleo, and gluten-free.

Times:

Preparation 15 min

Cooking 15 min

Total 30 min

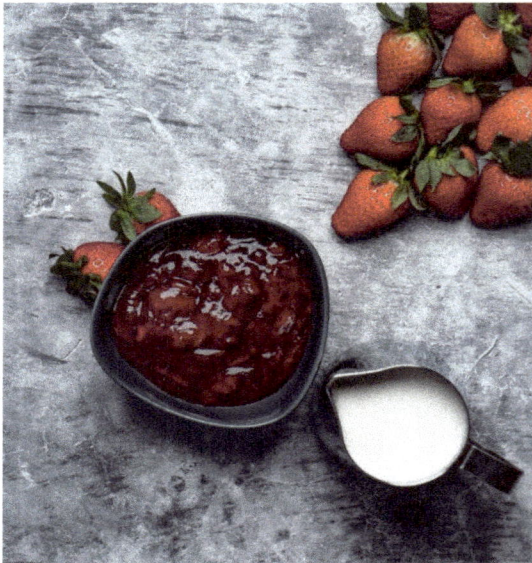

For 1 person:

Nutritional values

Calories 16

Net Carbohydrates 1.4 gr

Fats 0.5 gr

Protein 0.3 gr

MATERIALS

4 glass jars of 125 gr or 2 jars of 250 gr
with lids No stick pan

INGREDIENTS

500 gr of fresh or frozen strawberries

100 gr of erythritol

50 grams of chia seeds

1 tablespoon of balsamic vinegar

This jam is perfect to gratify a sudden desire f
or sweet or as an accompaniment to pancakes or sponge cake.
Very easy to prepare, it can be kept up to two weeks in the
refrigerator, healthy and cheap, especially when compared to
equivalent supermarket products, and if desired it can be kept
for much longer, putting it in a bain-marie for 45 minutes,
creating a vacuum seal.

INSTRUCTIONS

Put all the ingredients in a non-stick pan with high sides, let it cook over low heat, checking the consistency from time to time, after about 15 minutes the mixture should have reached the right density.

Pour the still hot jam into glass jars, previously sterilized in boiling water and left to cool upside down.

Substituting strawberries this is a recipe for making jams with many other types of fruit.

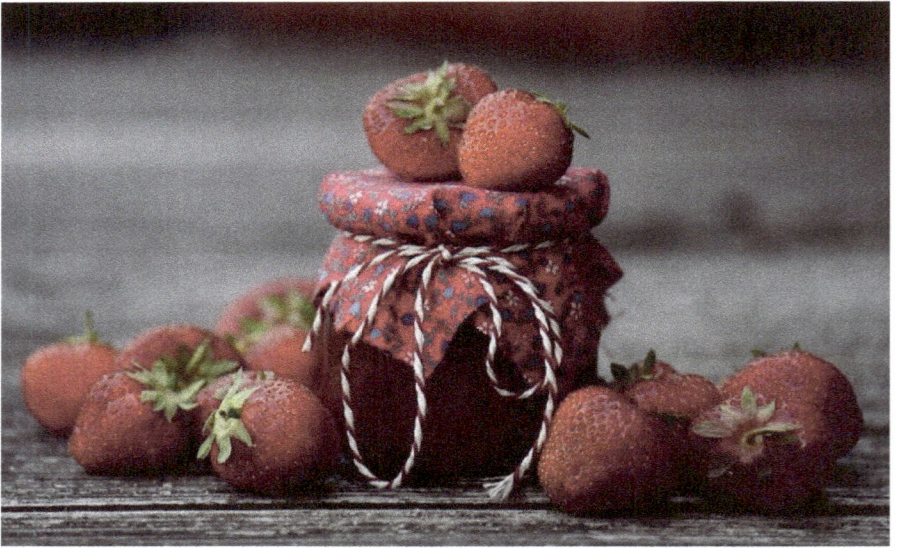

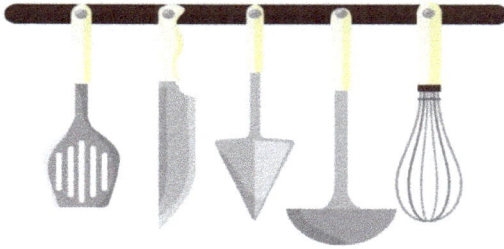

TART WITH CHOCOLATE AND COCONUT

This chocolate and coconut tart recipe is of medium difficulty, healthy, sugar-free and gluten-free but very tasty and beautiful to look at.

Take some time and enjoy the scents in making it, before the flavors.

Times:

Preparation 60 min

Cooking 30 min

Total 90 min

For 4/6 people

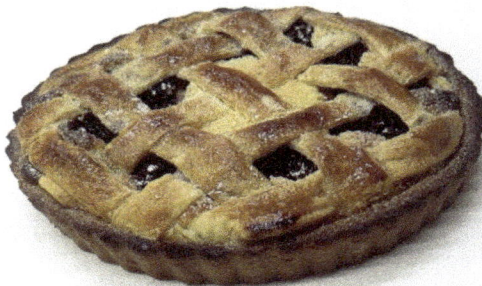

For 1 person:

Nutritional values

Calories 283

Carbohydrates 4 gr

Ratio 1.5 gr

Fats 24 gr

Protein 13.5 gr

MATERIALS

Mixer

1 cake pan 24/25 cm

1 small saucepan

1 bowl

INGREDIENTS

For the base

250 gr almond flour

50 gr erythritol

100 gr butter

2 eggs

For the stuffing

3 egg whites

50 gr erythritol

150 gr coconut turnips

For coverage

100 gr whipping cream

50 g 90% dark chocolate

INSTRUCTIONS

Blend the flour with the erythritol and the cold butter from the refrigerator in a blender, when it is all amalgamated, add the yolks while continuing to knead, to mix the mixture well.

Leave the mixture in the refrigerator for 30 minutes, then put it in the pan with a diameter of about 24 cm, after having greased or oiled it.

Heat the egg whites and erythritol in a bain-marie until the latter has dissolved completely, remove it from the heat and add the coconut, mixing the mixture.

Fill the base with the filling and bake in a ventilated oven for 30 minutes at 180 degrees.

Heat the cream, be very careful it shouldn't boil and melt the chocolate.

Pour the mixture over the cake.

Leave in the refrigerator for at least an hour.

Serve cold.

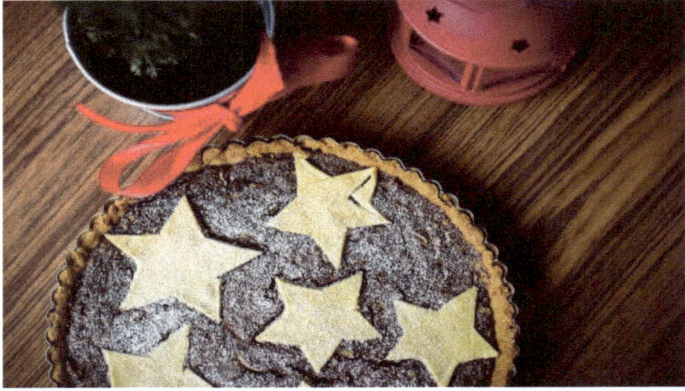

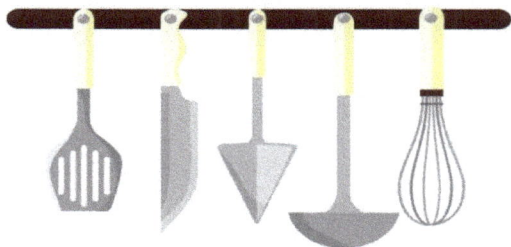

ALMOND AND LEMON GRAPE CAKE

This is a recipe for a truly special, fragrant and very soft cake, gluten-free, lactose-free, butter-free and sugar-free, therefore perfect for gratifying the taste without affecting the rules of the ketogenic diet.

Times:

Preparation 15 min

Cooking 40 min

Total 55 min

For 6 people

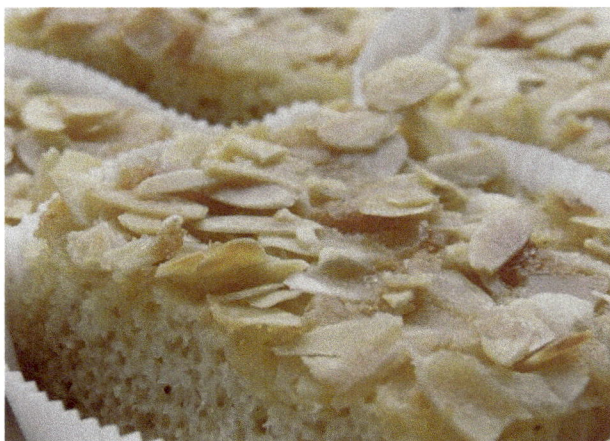

For 1 person:

Nutritional values

Calories 258

Carbohydrates 4.6 gr

Ratio 1.5

Fats 20 gr

Protein 11.7 gr

MATERIALS

Electric whips

20 cm diameter cake pan

INGREDIENTS

100 gr almond flour or finely chopped almonds

100 gr fine corn flour for cakes

or other flour (1, 0, 00)

50 gr rice flour

50 gr corn starch or potato starch

1 egg

100 gr of egg whites

180 gr vegetable or soy cream

120 gr erythritol or 100 gr cane or normal

or coconut sugar, or 60 gr stevia

1 lemon (zest) or lemon flavoring

200 gr grapes

1 pinch of baking soda

1 sachet of baking powder

INSTRUCTIONS

Cut the grapes in half by carefully removing all the seeds, put the seedless grapes on one side and whisk the egg in a bowl together with the egg white and the chosen sweetener, until the mixture is light and fluffy. add the vegetable cream, always continuing to whip.

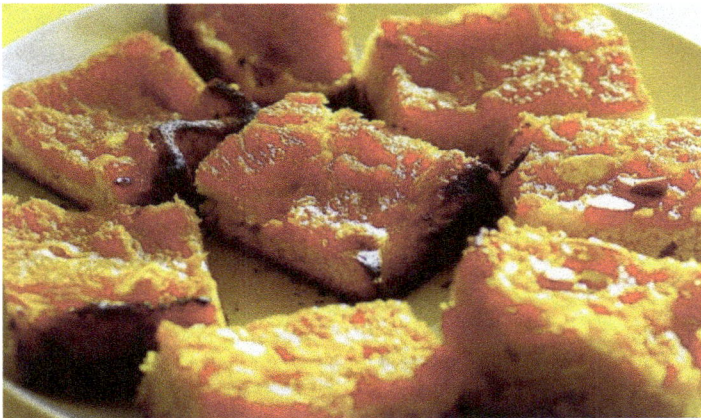

In a separate bowl, add the flours to the yeast sachet, also add a pinch of baking soda, always continuing to mix well, so that the flours are mixed evenly and above all without lumps. Add the grated zest of a lemon (or the aroma) to the flour, add the dry ingredients to the liquids a couple of tablespoons at a time, little by little, continuing to mix to keep the mixture homogeneous. Now add 3/4 of the grapes prepared previously to the mixture and incorporate it well into the mixture with a spatula.

Pour the mixture into the previously greased or oiled and floured cake pan or lined with parchment paper, decorate the surface of the mixture as desired by making drawings with the remaining grapes.

Put in a ventilated or static oven at 180 ° / 170 ° degrees for about 45 minutes, to see if it is cooked well the toothpick rule applies, a rule for all baked desserts, use a toothpick, pierce the cake and if it comes out without nothing attached means that it is ready.

Serve cold or just warm.

The cake can be frozen and consumed later, defrosting it in the microwave or naturally. It can be kept unfrozen after cooking, Well, covered for 2 or 3 days.

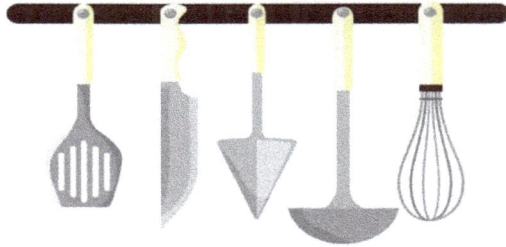

ORANGE AND CINNAMON CAKE

This cake is made in less than 1 hour and with medium
difficulty, particularly soft and fragrant, very suitable for
breakfast or at all times of the day when you want
to have an extra gear.

Times:

Preparation 10 min

Cooking 40 min

Total 50 min

For 6 people

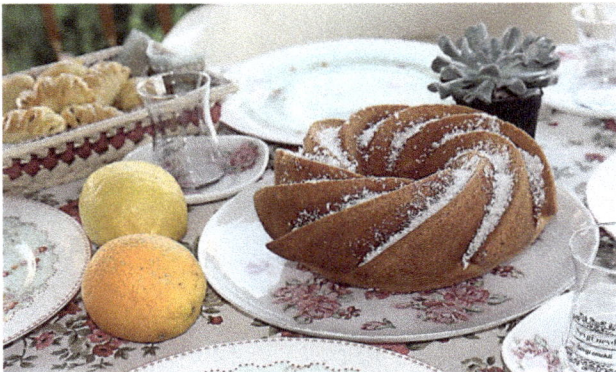

For 1 person:

Nutritional values

Calories 356

Carbohydrates 12.5 gr

Ratio 1.93 gr

Fat 54 gr

Protein 14 gr

Fiber 14.5 gr

Sugars 0.5 gr

MATERIALS

1 24 cm hinged cake pan

(the edge of the

pan can be removed)

Electric whisks, mixer or planetary

1 sieve

1 bowl

INGREDIENTS

120 gr wholemeal flour

40 gr coconut flour

40 gr corn starch or potato starch

16 gr baking powder

q.s. cinnamon

3 egg

125 gr 0% fat Greek yogurt

20 ml coconut or seed oil

(5 ml is a teaspoon)

90 ml orange juice

45 gr stevia or 120 gr erythritol

or 75 gr cane sugar

1 tsp organic orange peel

2/3 slices of orange to decorate

INSTRUCTIONS

Whip the egg with the granular sweetener you have chosen until the mixture is light and fluffy, continuing to mix, add the oil and yogurt, then the juice and orange zest. Add the sifted flours together with the baking powder and cinnamon to the frothy mixture. Sprinkle the bottom of the pan previously lined with parchment paper or greased and floured paper, with granular sweetener (truvia or erythritol) or with cane or coconut sugar or at most normal sugar, with cinnamon.

Sugar and cinnamon will caramelize the surface of the cake.

Now put the orange slices cut 3/4 mm thick on the bottom of the pan to cover the entire circumference of the mold, pour the mixture over the orange slices so as to cover them and bake in the preheated oven at 180 degrees to 5 minutes, and cook for another 40 minutes or so.

It is important that the surface of the cake is golden, if you have any doubles use the toothpick trick *.

* if the cake is cooked nothing will stick to the toothpick.

After the toothpick test and proven cooking with the golden surface of the cake, remove it from the oven and let it cool.

Turn your cake upside down on a plate so that the side with the orange slices faces up.

Now decorate as you like, if you want with more cinnamon.

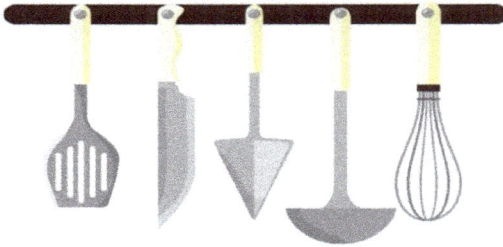

MUFFIN BANANA AND PECAN

For our recipes these ingredients and nutritional values are fundamental, read carefully when you shop, all of this is very important for our health. Avoid foods that contain additives that have only decorative / aesthetic purposes, because they are absolutely useless for the quality of your kitchen and instead harmful. On the other hand, there are flavors with which we can replace non-ketogenic ingredients, such as fruit with a lot of sugar or caramel.

Times:

Preparation 60 min

Cooking 30 min

Total 90 min

For 12 muffins

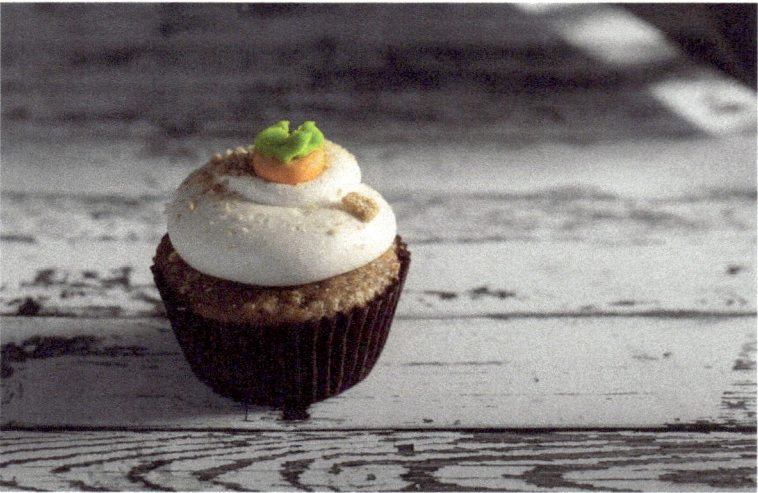

For 1 muffin:

Nutritional values

Calories 210

Carbohydrates 1.47 gr

Ratio 2.46 gr

Fats 19.09 gr

Protein 6.48 gr

MATERIALS

Electric whips

1 bowl

12 paper or silicone cups

INGREDIENTS

135 gr almond flour

90 gr Dieta medicale Pasta flour

30 gr erythritol

60 gr butter

75 gr fresh cream

3 medium egg (55gr)

12 gr instant yeast

60 drops banana aroma Bulkpowders Liquiflav

60 gr pecans of which 12 whole kernels for decoration and all the rest chopped.

INSTRUCTIONS

In this recipe the amount of erythritol used is very small because the Liquiflav flavors are sweetened with sucralose, mix all the ingredients with an electric whisk, leaving the whole kernels on one side. Divide everything by pouring the mixture into 12 muffin cups, the paper ones of many colors are very nice.

Put a whole kernel inside each muffin, pushing it a little inside, inside the dough, because as it rises in the oven it will rise again and will serve to decorate. Bake the muffins in a preheated convection oven for 5 minutes at 160 ° degrees and bake for another 20 minutes. The coloring contained in the aroma will give a pleasant golden appearance to the surface of the muffins.

Serve them hot / lukewarm.

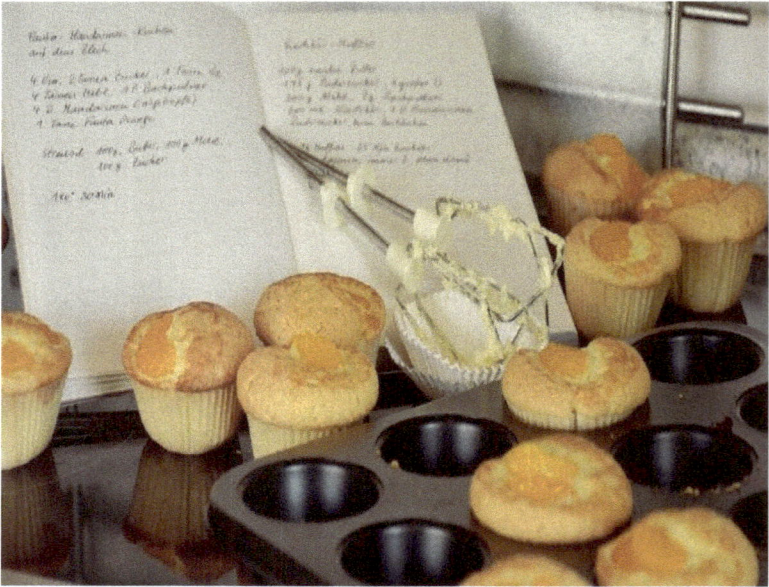

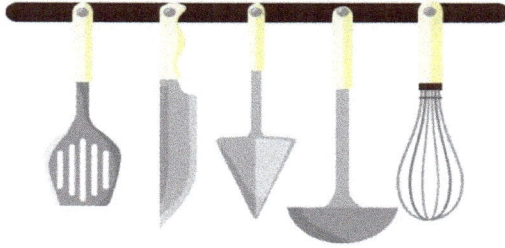

BASIL, STRAWBERRY AND LEMON CAKE

Making this recipe well might seem simple, but it is not at all like that, as all simple recipes should not be underestimated and as you well know, this rule is especially true for cooking desserts that must be particularly taken care of in every phase. For example, the egg whites must be whipped to perfection and all the ingredients mixed with delicacy and love.

Times:

Preparation 10 min

Cooking 50 min

Total 60 min

For 6 people

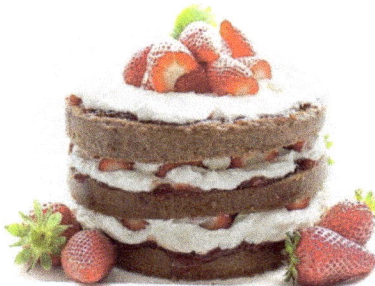

For 1 person:

Nutritional values

Calories 240

Carbohydrates 15 gr

Fat 6 gr

Protein 30 gr

MATERIALS

1 cake pan of 16 cm

Electric whips

2 Bowls

INGREDIENTS

20 gr brown rice flour

10 gr corn starch

35 gr coconut flour

20 gr oat flour

25 gr oat flakes flavored with lemon
cream or other normal oats and ½ lemon zest

½ sachet of baking powder or 1 teaspoon
of bicarbonate and lemon juice or 1 sachet
of hydrolithin and water or cream
of tartar and 1 pinch of bicarbonate

40 gr stevia or other natural sweetener

1 egg

50 gr egg white

50 gr apple pulp

15 gr coconut oil

100/130 ml coconut milk or
other vegetable milk

200 gr strawberries

10 basil leaves

½ lemon zest use the zest of a whole
lemon if you are not using flavored oat flakes

Depending on the flours used, the dough could be more or less dense, we recommend using 100 ml of milk more and adding the rest if the dough is too thick.

INSTRUCTIONS

Preheat the oven, preferably ventilated, at 180 degrees for 10 minutes, in a bowl add the flour with yeast, stevia and lemon zest. In another bowl, instead, combine the egg, egg white, apple pulp, coconut oil and coconut milk.

Mix the liquid ingredients well with an electric whisk or by hand and add the dry ingredients a little at a time, more or less 3 times, taking care to incorporate well to obtain a mixture without lumps, now add the strawberries and the basil cut into small pieces.

An important tip: chop the basil with your hands and not with a knife to prevent it from oxidizing. If you do not use yeast, now add the hydrolithin and let it react with a little water, or the baking soda with a few drops of lemon, mix well, making sure the foam disappears, so that the taste is not bitter. Pour the mixture into a pan lined with parchment paper and bake at 180 degrees for 50/60 minutes, then use the toothpick test.

The cake keeps well, moist and soft for 3 or 4 days.

Best if covered with a cake bell, and before eating it is recommended to heat a little in the microwave oven.

It is possible to freeze it in single portions by cutting it into slices.

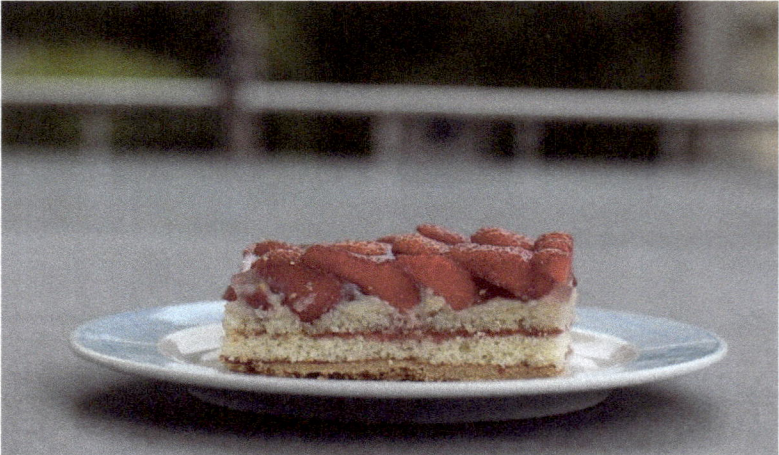

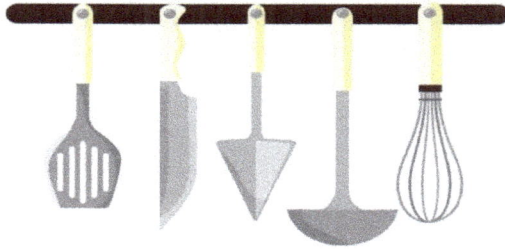

WAFFLE WITH ALMOND FLOUR

This is a recipe in a keto and low-carb version of waffles, which obviously do not need to be presented, because they are well-known and appreciated sweets both sweet and savory, combined with any type of food. The original recipe is a Belgian specialty that is now famous all over the world. This recipe is the ketogenic version of sweet waffles, which are equally delicious despite being an adapted version of the original recipe and which are also very popular with those who have no restrictions on carbohydrate consumption.

Times:

Preparation 10 min

Cooking 50 min

Total 60 min

For 6 people

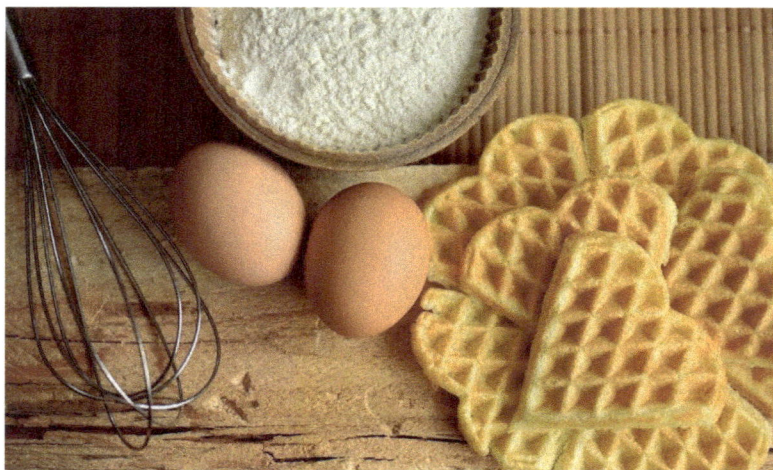

For 1 person:

Nutritional values

Calories 299

Carbohydrates 1.31 gr

Sugars 1.4 gr

Fats 17.4 gr

Protein 6.8 gr

Ratio 2.13 gr

MATERIALS

Electric whips

1 baking dish 24/26 cm

1 small saucepan

1 Cylindrical container

or glass great

Waffle toaster

INGREDIENTS

115 gr almond flour

10 gr oat fiber

40 gr erythritol

10 gr tilts

3 medium eggs

150 gr fresh cream

15 gr melted but not hot butter

vanilla or vanillin

INSTRUCTIONS

This waffle recipe is yeast-free, the eggs still give the waffles a leavened and crunchy texture. Preheat the machine, put all the ingredients in a large cylindrical glass and mix with an electric whisk at medium speed or by hand, to form a fluid mixture, pour the mixture into the molds of the machine until they are almost full and close the lid. Normally averaged with several machines, waffles cook in about 5-7 minutes after closing the lid. Be very careful not to pass the correct cooking point and do not overcook them to prevent the erythritol from turning dark, this is not good for your health. Remember that the waffles are cooked more below than above, take the first waffles from the molds when they have the right degree of cooking, continue following to pour the mixture into the molds, always mixing the batter before pouring it.

Serve hot or lukewarm accompanied by ice cream, fruit or whatever you prefer,
they are quite soft for this reason they are also good on their own, or with a little low-carb jam and a spoonful of whipped cream.

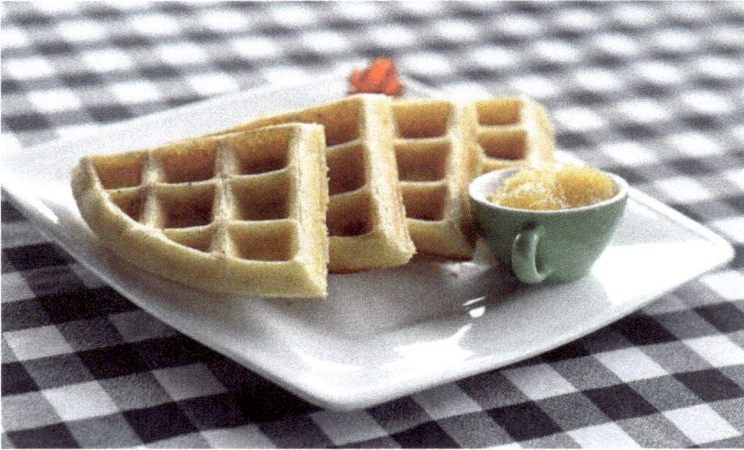

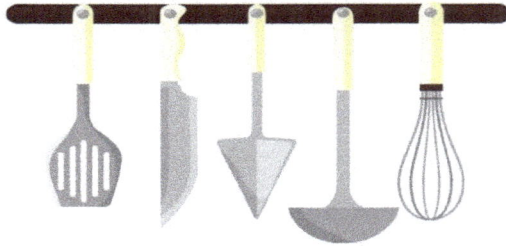

PANCAKES WITH ALMOND FLOUR

This is a recipe to have a good alternative to classic pancakes, they are very simple to make and ideal for breakfast, obviously keto-friendly.

Times:

Preparation 15 min

Cooking 15 min

Total 30 min

For 6 people

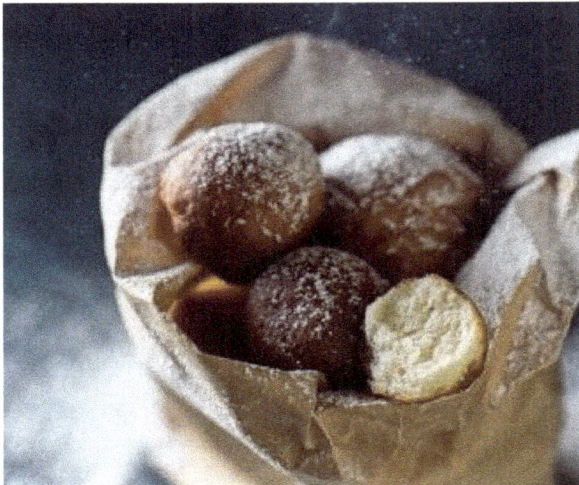

For 1 person (2 pancakes):

Nutritional values

Calories 219

Carbohydrates 11 gr

Fat 29 gr

Protein 14 gr

MATERIALS

Electric whips

1 Non-stick pan or specific for pancakes
with 4 internal molds

1 bowl

1 Cylindrical container or large glass

INGREDIENTS

115 gr almond flour

10 gr oat fiber

5 gr of yeast for sweets

40 gr erythritol

10 gr tilts

3 medium eggs

150 gr fresh cream

15 gr melted but not hot butter

vanilla or vanillin

INSTRUCTIONS

This recipe is particularly quick and simple, the pancakes can be stored in the refrigerator for up to 5 days, they are perfect as breakfast or as a snack. The preparation is the same as the waffles in the recipe you find above, just add 5 grams of baking powder to the mixture to make
the pancakes more puffy and fluffy.
To have pancakes of the same size it would be perfect to use a special non-stick pan that has four round parts, where you will pour the batter that will not go all over the place and the pancakes are all the same.
Serve hot or lukewarm with zero syrup or a splash of unsweetened whipped cream.

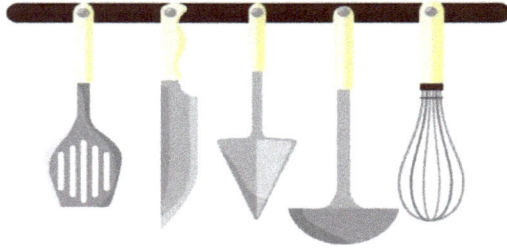

PLUMCAKE WITH PEACHES AND CHOCOLATE DROPS

This is the recipe for making a soft plum cake with peaches and chocolate chips, delicious and ideal for a snack or for breakfast, accompanied by a cup of coffee.

Times:

Preparation 10 min

Cooking 45 min

Total 55 min

For 10 servings

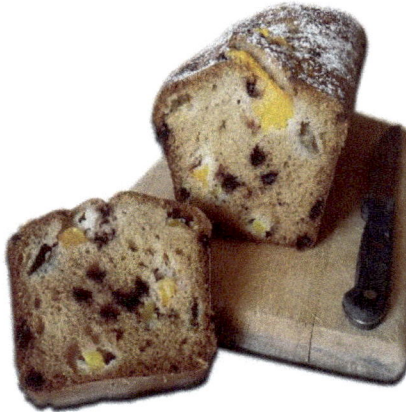

For 1 person:

Nutritional values

Calories 132

Carbohydrates 1.27 gr

Ratio 2.46

Fats 19.09 gr

Protein 6.49 gr

MATERIALS

1 25 cm loaf pan

Electric or hand whips

2 Bowls

INGREDIENTS

200 g type 0 or 1 or 00 flour

35 g coconut flour

2 eggs

60 g fruit puree or 1 other egg

100 ml vegetable or rice milk

15 g seed oil or coconut oil or EVO oil

1 pinch of baking soda

1 sachet of baking powder

2 small peaches or 1 large

30 g chocolate chips without sugar

200g erythritol or 70g stevia

or other granular sugar substitute

INSTRUCTIONS

Preheat the oven to 180 degrees for about 10 minutes, peel the peaches and cut them into pieces that are not too small, whip the eggs together with the sweetener until the mixture is light and fluffy. In another bowl, combine the flours with the baking powder and baking soda, mixing well so that all the ingredients mix well. Add the flours to the egg mixture in two times and mix thoroughly, always stirring making sure that the mixture is frothy and fluid, add the milk gently gradually while continuing to mix. Then add the oil and continue to mix carefully you will get a smooth mixture, not too liquid and without lumps.

Now add the chocolate chips to the dough and continue to mix this time with a spoon or a whisk so that they are evenly distributed. Pour the mixture into the loaf pan lined with parchment paper, or oiled or buttered, add the chopped peaches on the surface then press a little and lightly so that they enter the mixture.

Place in the oven and cook for about 45 minutes, always checking until the toothpick test is done.

Be careful to put the pieces of peach last, so that they also remain on the surface.

Serve hot or warm.

For breakfast it will be perfect accompanied by a yogurt or a good cappuccino.

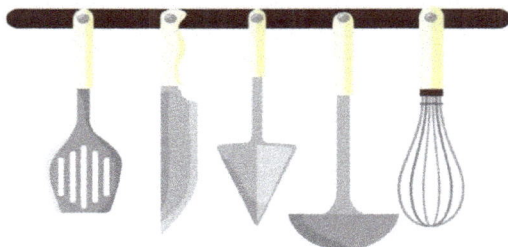

LEMON CAKE

This super-fast lemon dessert is a single-serving dessert that cooks in the microwave in less than two minutes, for a total of 5 minutes with preparation.

This single-serving dessert takes its lemon flavor from both the juice and the zest, the juice makes the dough very moist to be eaten with a spoon, the lemon zest, on the other hand, enhances its flavor.

Times:

Preparation 3 min

Cooking 2 min

Total 5 min

For 4 baking cups

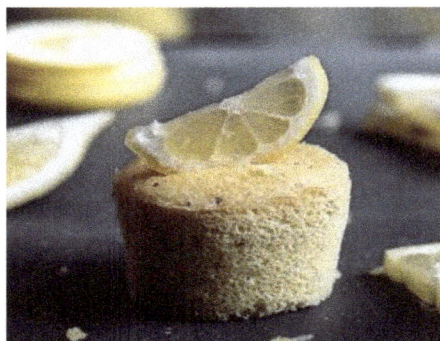

For 1 person / baking cup:

Nutritional values

Calories 128

Carbohydrates 7.8 gr

Ratio 2.46 gr

Fat 3 gr

Protein 3.4 gr

MATERIALS

4 microwave-safe baking cups with
a diameter of 8/9 cm,
preferably in glass or oven ceramic.

INGREDIENTS

180 gr almond flour

20 gr of powdered erythriol

1 teaspoon of baking powder

1/3 teaspoon of salt

3 tablespoons of fresh lemon

20 gr of melted butter

1 tablespoon of fresh lemon zest

INSTRUCTIONS

Mix the dry ingredients first and then add the wet ones, as
sweetener we have chosen erythritol, but you can use any other
sweetener with zero calories, the important thing is that you

sweeten in the same way, in this recipe the powdered sweetener works better than the granular one.

Put the mixture in the various cups, if they are found in all ways, glass and ceramic are preferable, given the high temperatures and cook in the microwave for 2 minutes each. This sweet can be served hot or cold, decorated with a slice of lemon or with a little sugar-free whipped cream, great as a snack.

Each cake takes about 1 1/2 minutes to cook, but the more cakes they cook together in the microwave, the more you need to increase the cooking time.

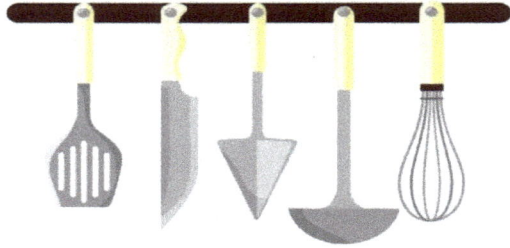

ICE CREAM CAKE

The cream ice cream cake is a delicious keto and gluten-free cake, to be served cold, the cake is reminiscent of the famous cream heart ice cream croissant.

A very simple summer dessert to prepare, low in carbohydrates to keep in the freezer, to eat it just keep it at room temperature for about 10/12 minutes, after which we can easily cut it and serve it.

The cake is based on a pancakes with coconut and hazelnuts, with a very greedy flavor.

Times:

Preparation 40 min

Freezing 120/180 minutes

Total 160/220 min

For 6/8 people

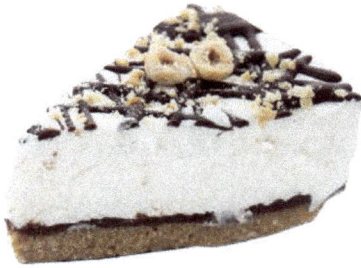

For 1 person:

Nutritional values

Calories 210

Carbohydrates 1.27 gr

Ratio 2.46 gr

Fats 18.07 gr

Protein 6.49 gr

MATERIALS

1 pan of 20 cm

1 20 cm springform mold

Film

Greaseproof paper

Planetary or electric whisks

2 Bowls

INGREDIENTS

500 ml of unsweetened fresh liquid
whipping cream

250 gr Mascarpone

3 and a half tablespoons of fructose

or stevia or erythritol to evaluate the quantities

1 sachet of vanillin or seeds of half a vanilla bean

80 gr of dark chocolate from 72% upwards

25 gr of clarified butter

100 gr of whole toasted hazelnuts

For the pancakes:

3 medium eggs

2 tablespoons of fructose or 2 and

a half tablespoons of coconut sugar (preferable)

1 teaspoon of fine coconut flour

2 tablespoons of hazelnut flour

1 tablespoon of dried grated coconut or turnips'

2 teaspoons of unsweetened cocoa

2 tablespoons of coconut oil

a pinch of baking soda for food

or the tip of a teaspoon of baking powder

a knob of butter for the pan

INSTRUCTIONS

Prepare the base with the mixture for the pancake, in a small bowl put all the ingredients together, mixing by hand or with electric whisk at low speed and mix well, then pour everything into the pan where you have previously melted a small knob of butter or a little bit of oil.

When the base is cooked, turn it, check it by adjusting to the color that must be golden, and complete the cooking, then put it on one side to cool.

Line the springform pan with parchment paper on the base and foil on the edges.

In a planetary mixer or with a bowl with an electric mixer, whip the cream with the vanilla, mascarpone and sweetener of your choice, when you have finished whipping the mixture, you can begin to assemble the cake, placing the large pancake on the base of the pan and pouring it over. the mascarpone and cream, smooth and level the cream, then cover with plastic wrap and put it in the freezer for a few hours, at least 6 hours.

After a perfect day, if you are in a hurry it will take 6 hours, you can remove it from the freezer and from the mold, put it in a serving dish and complete it by putting the melted dark chocolate and hazelnuts.

For the chocolate and hazelnut coating:

Lightly chop some hazelnuts in order to have both whole and chopped.

Melt the dark chocolate with the butter and pour it on the cake starting from the center and then reaching the edges trying to cover everything, help yourself with a spoon or a small spatula.

Finally, add the hazelnuts to the chocolate and put the cake back in the freezer.

Before serving it should be kept for a while letting it rest for about ten minutes so that it can be cut easily and it will be ready to be eaten. The cream ice cream cake can also be prepared without the base, therefore without the large pancake, simpler, or it can be replaced with a more delicious base made with chopped hazelnuts.

Note:

To finish, put the cake in the freezer for a minimum of six hours before adding the chocolate and hazelnuts, even better freezing it for a whole day.

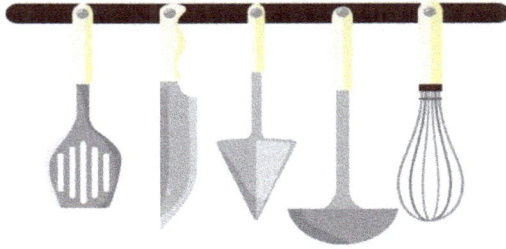

COCONUT, CHERRIES AND CHOCOLATE PANCAKES

The Pancakes in this recipe are low carb, gluten-free, lactose-free and sugar-free.

Tasty and suitable for all those who follow a low-carbohydrate diet, such as the Paleo diet or the Ketogenic diet.

Also perfect for those with blood sugar problems, for celiacs and lactose intolerant.

Times:

Preparation 20 min

Cooking 15 min

Total 160/220 min

For 10 pancakes

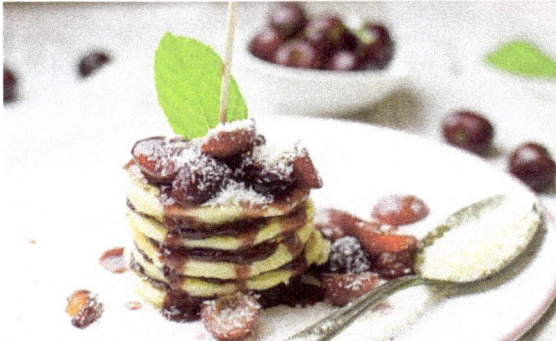

For 1 pancake:

Nutritional values

Calories 242

Carbohydrates 5.8 gr

Fat 1.8 gr

Protein 4.1 gr

MATERIALS

Electric whips

1 bowl

1 small pan

INGREDIENTS

2 large organic eggs

4 tablespoons of dried grated

coconut or turnips'

cinnamon to taste

1 1/2 tablespoons of coconut oil

250 gr of cherries

2/3 squares of dark chocolate

from 75% upwards

1 teaspoon of honey or sweetener

of your choice (optional)

INSTRUCTIONS

Start by washing and drying the cherries thoroughly, put some whole cherries on one side to garnish the dish and the others cut them in half, taking care to remove the core, put the chopped cherries in a small pan with a little ghee butter and a teaspoon. of honey, 3 tablespoons of water and a pinch of cinnamon, put the pan on the heat and let them cook with the lid on for about 4 minutes, over medium heat, stirring often, making sure that it does not dry too much,
once ready, remove them from the heat and keep them to one side.
Now let's move on to preparing the pancakes, separate the yolks from the whites and whisk the latter until stiff peaks, add the coconut turnips to the yolks, 1/3 teaspoon of cinnamon, coconut oil and mix everything together,
now gently add the egg whites to the mixture of yolks and coconut,
let's cook them in a pan with very little coconut oil or ghee butter,
we will prepare 4, for each pancake the amount of dough will be about 1 and a half tablespoons.
Once ready we put them in a nice dish and alternate them with sautéed cherries, finally we will add fresh cherries and dark chocolate flakes or chopped.
It is possible to use other types of fruit such as strawberries and raspberries.

If you want to speed up the preparation, I recommend serving the pancakes with sugar-free cherry jam and using fresh cherries as a garnish to eat plain.

If you are super greedy, you can melt the dark chocolate and pour it over the pancakes.

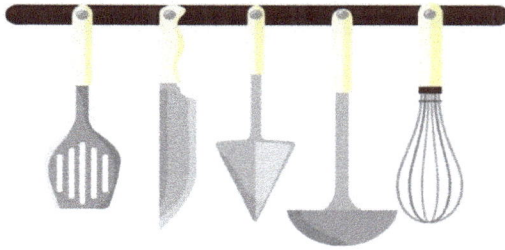

SOFT APRICOT TART

The soft apricot tart, low-carb, that is, low in carbohydrates, gluten-free, lactose-free and paleo is a light and digestible cake. Low-carb desserts are increasingly popular and well-known, and it is also perfect for those who follow a Keto diet.

Times:

Preparation 20 min

Cooling down 2 hours

Total 2 hours and 20 min

For 6/8 people

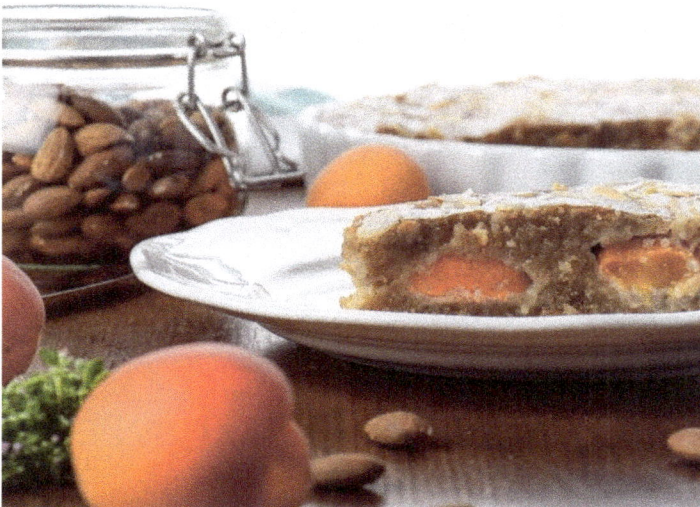

For 1 slice:

Nutritional values

Calories 242

Carbohydrates 24 gr

Fats 16 gr

Protein 7 gr

MATERIALS

1 Filling mold

Mixer or food processor

1 small saucepan

INGREDIENTS

4 large eggs

40 gr of whole unpeeled almonds

75 gr dried or rapé grated coconut

25 grams of fine coconut flour

4 tablespoons of coconut oil

5 apricots

35 grams of coconut sugar

half a sachet of cream of tartar or baking powder

1 teaspoon of cinnamon or 1 sachet of vanillin

butter and coconut flour for the smart

26/28 cm mold with low edge

For the apricot jelly:

12 apricots

half an apple

(optional) 2 tablespoons of

coconut sugar or 1 large tablespoon of honey

5 gr of isinglass or gelatin

the juice of half a lemon

6 Apricots as a cake decoration

INSTRUCTIONS

For this recipe, grease the filling mold and flour it with fine coconut flour, turn on the convection oven at 170 ° degrees and preheat it for 5 minutes.

Put the almonds in the mixer or food processor, chop them well until they are reduced to flour together with the shredded coconut and the coconut flour, then add all the other ingredients except the yeast and mix well and thoroughly, now you can also add the yeast, incorporate it well and pour it all into the 26/28 cm filling mold, put it to cook in a ventilated oven at 170 degrees for about 20 minutes.

While the soft tart is in the oven you can start preparing the apricot jelly, immediately soak the isinglass and pour the apricots and half an apple previously cleaned and cut into other small pieces, lemon juice, the chosen sweetener and purée, at this point cook over high heat until it starts to boil, then add the well squeezed isinglass, mix everything well and set it aside to cool, and do not use it until it is lukewarm.

Now you can take the cake out of the oven, let it cool before removing it from the mold, when the cake is cold we can pour the still warm fruit jelly into the center of the hollow and put it in the fridge promptly.

After about 2 hours move on to the decoration with the apricots cut into a fan or as you prefer with your imagination.

So it will be perfect to be served.

Note:

We can also prepare this cake with many other types of seasonal fruit, we could use strawberries, peaches, figs but in this case we will not add sugars.

It can be kept in the refrigerator, take it out 5/10 minutes before eating it.

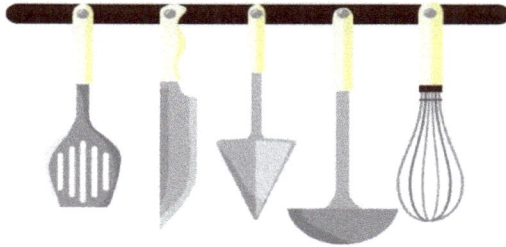

COCONUT AND HAZELNUT PANCAKE

This recipe is super simple, super quick, super Keto, super low-carb, and invariably super yummy.

Times:

Preparation 10 min

Cooking 15 min

Total 35 min

For 10 pancakes

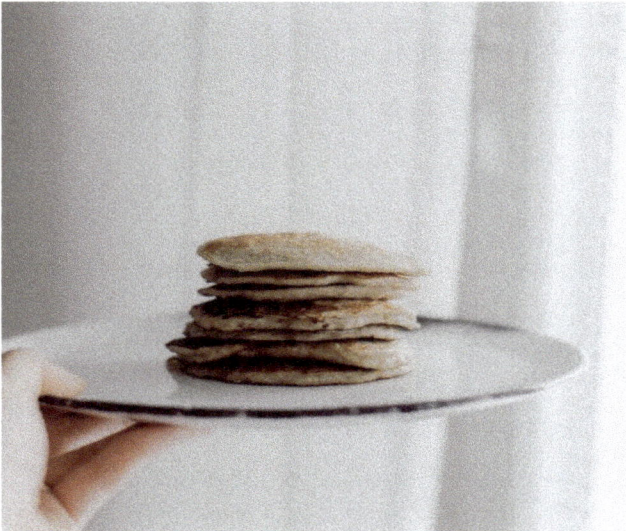

For 1 pancake:

Nutritional values

Calories 90

Carbohydrates 7.5 gr

Fat 1.5 gr

Protein 12 gr

MATERIALS

1 bowl

1 small non-stick pan with a diameter of about 12 cm

INGREDIENTS

3 medium eggs

2 tablespoons of fructose or 2 and a half

tablespoons of coconut sugar (preferable)

1 teaspoon of fine coconut flour

2 tablespoons of hazelnut flour

1 sachet of yeast

1 glass of milk

1 tablespoon of dried grated coconut or turnips'

2 teaspoons of unsweetened cocoa

2 tablespoons of coconut oil

1 pinch of baking soda or the tip

of a teaspoon of baking powder

1 pinch of salt

1 drop of oil or 1 knob of butter for the pan

INSTRUCTIONS

To make the pancakes, put all the dry ingredients, that is the
three types of flour, fructose, a pinch of yeast and a pinch of salt
in a large bowl and mix well, by hand or with electric whisk
then add the eggs and a little to the turn the milk, and the rest
of the ingredients, working everything until the mixture is
creamy and fairly homogeneous.

Take a small non-stick pan, about 12 cm in diameter, and
grease the bottom just slightly with a drop of oil or butter.
Heat it, then take 2 generous spoons of dough and pour them
into the center of the pan, the dough must cover the entire
bottom.

As soon as the pancake takes on color, turn it over and cook it
on the other side.

Continue like this until the dough is used up.

Stuffed to your taste, sugar-free cream and fruit or jam.

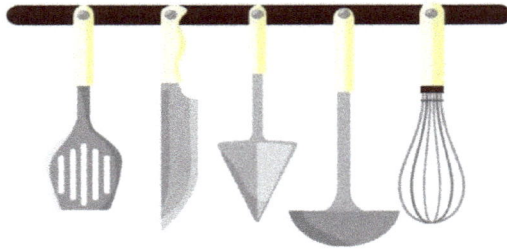

DONUTS

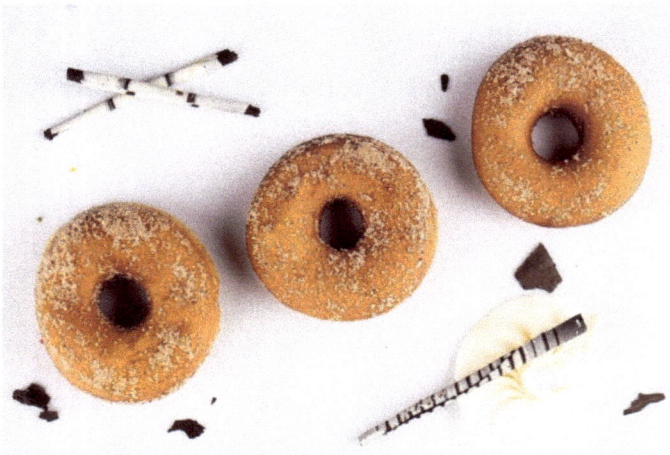

Times:

Preparation 40 min

Freezing 120/180 minutes

Total 160/220 min

For 6/8 people

For 1 person:

Nutritional values

Calories 70

Carbohydrates 4.5 gr

Fat 2 gr

Protein 5 gr

MATERIALS

Electric whips

1 baking sheet

Small saucepan

INGREDIENTS

3 cups of mascarpone cream

4 tablespoons of cream cheese

1.1 / 2 cup of almond flour

2 tablespoons of xanthan gum

2 eggs

1 sachet of instant yeast for savory

2 tablespoons of butter

2 tablespoons of sweetener

INSTRUCTIONS

Preheat the oven, preferably ventilated, at 180 degrees for about 10 minutes, at the same time dissolve the yeast in a glass with a cup of warm water.

In a bowl put the almond flour, the xanthan gum and mix carefully, add the eggs, the melted butter, the previously diluted yeast and mix and mix everything, finally add the mascarpone and the cream cheese and knead well until 'you will not get a soft to the touch, smooth and homogeneous dough.

Now form regular balls and delicately make a central hole for each ball, so as to make donuts, place the donuts on a baking sheet with a sheet of parchment paper and bake for about 10/12 minutes.

Remove the donuts from the oven only when they are golden. Serve them hot / lukewarm for breakfast or as a snack, accompanied by a fragrant coffee or freshly squeezed orange juice.

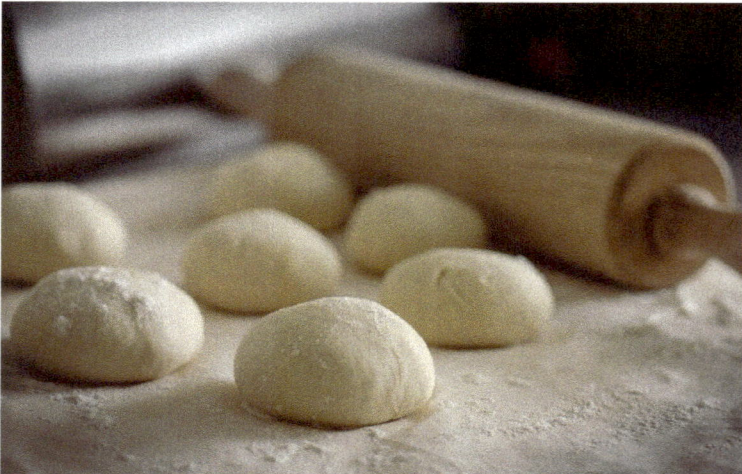

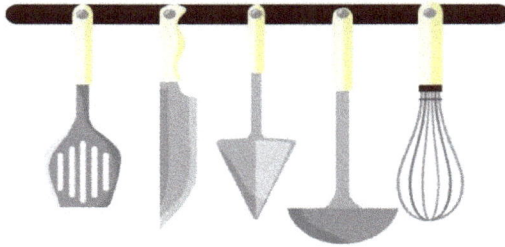

CHOCOLATE CAKE

This recipe for a ketogenic chocolate cake is an easy recipe to make, although not particularly greedy, but without sugar, without flour and without yeast, therefore perfect for appeasing the desire for sweet that often occurs within a ketogenic diet.

Times:

Preparation 20 min

Cooking 40 min

Total 60 min

For 6/8 people

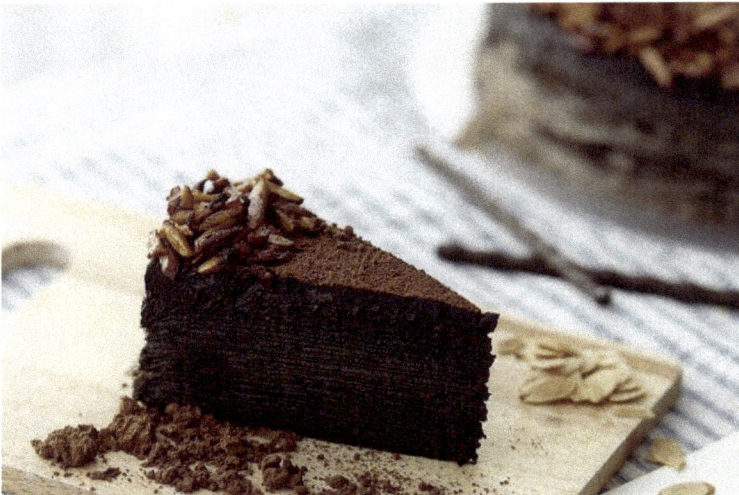

For 1 slice:

Nutritional values

Calories 250

Carbohydrates 3 gr

Sugars 4 gr

Fats 18.5 gr

Protein 13.5 gr

MATERIALS

Electric whips

1 hinged cake pan 25/25 cm

1 small saucepan

2 Bowls

INGREDIENTS

200 g of dark chocolate from 85% upwards

100 ml of extra virgin olive oil

3 eggs

200 grams of almond flour

2 tablespoons of unsweetened cocoa

Salt to taste.

white yogurt lean no and fresh fruit to decorate

INSTRUCTIONS

Start this recipe by taking 2 bowls and separate the yolks from the whites, in a bowl put the egg whites and whisk them until stiff adding a pinch of salt and in the other bowl the yolks, put the dark chocolate bars in a saucepan, start breaking them and melt them in a bain-marie. Beat the egg yolks with the olive oil and add the melted chocolate, almond flour and bitter cocoa. Mix and mix everything thoroughly with a wooden spoon, now add the whipped egg whites, mixing from top to bottom to incorporate them properly, when you have finished the mixture should be moist but compact.

Grease the bottom of a hinged cake pan and pour in all the mixture, bake in a ventilated oven for 30/40 minutes at 170 ° degrees, when the cake is cooked, if in doubt the toothpick test is always valid, remove it from the oven and do it cool down. When the cake is cold, you can gently open the hinged cake pan and place the chocolate cake on a serving plate or cake stand and decorate with a layer of yogurt and fresh fruit, such as strawberries, raspberries or blueberries.

Ready to eat.

It can be kept in the fridge for about 4 days.

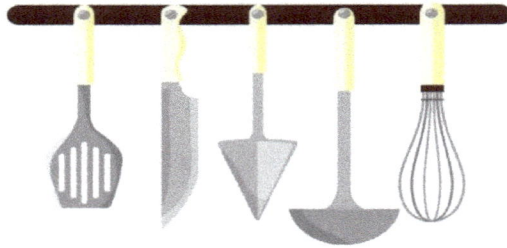

HONEY SHORT PASTRY

Times:

Preparation 30 min

Cooling in the fridge 30 min

Cooking 10 min

Total 70 min

For 40 biscuits or for 2 tarts

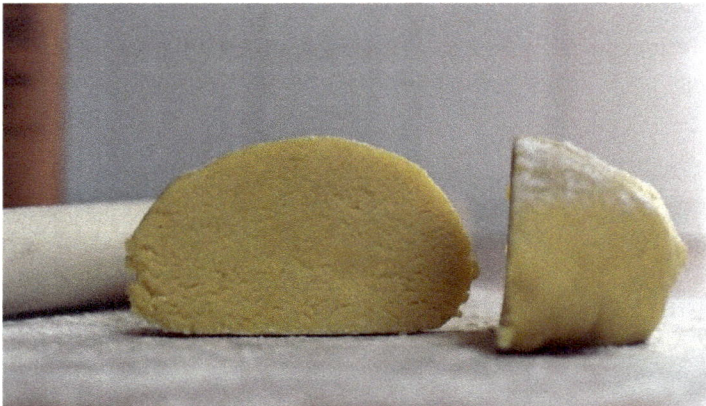

For 1 person:

Nutritional values

Calories 174

Carbohydrates 12.7 gr

Fat 12 gr

Protein 16 gr

MATERIALS

1 bowl

Film

Oven pan

Greaseproof paper

Coppapasta or cookie cutters

INGREDIENTS

340 gr Mix of gluten-free flours for pies and biscuits

or 200 gr rice flour and 140g corn flour

100 gr Coconut oil

120 gr Honey

3 eggs

q.s. Vanilla flavor or favorite flavor,

you can also use cinnamon

1/2 sachet sachet yeast for sweets

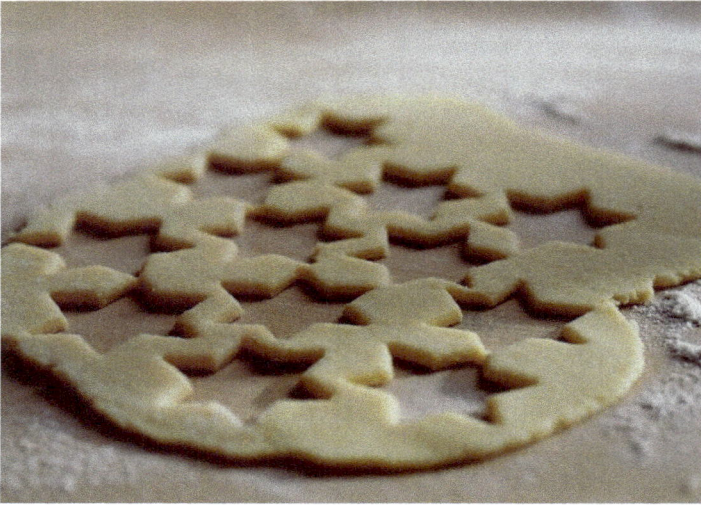

INSTRUCTIONS

Preheat the oven to 180 ° degrees for 15 minutes, in the meantime create a fountain with the flour and yeast inside a bowl and gradually add the eggs, coconut oil, honey to the center of the fountain. and the vanilla flavor.

Knead vigorously by hand until you get a solid and at the same time easily workable dough. Wrap the mixture in plastic wrap and put it to rest for 30 minutes in the fridge. After 30 minutes, take the mixture from the fridge and roll it out with a rolling pin, after which you can have fun giving the most varied shapes with a pastry cutter or cookie cutters.

When you have finished bake on a baking sheet with parchment paper at 180 degrees for about 10 minutes or remove them from the oven when they are golden brown.

Serve them lukewarm.

Note:

For the two-tone cocoa short crust pastry recipe just add 1
tablespoon of bitter cocoa to the short crust pastry stick,
kneading thoroughly until the cocoa
is well incorporated,
before putting it in the fridge to rest.

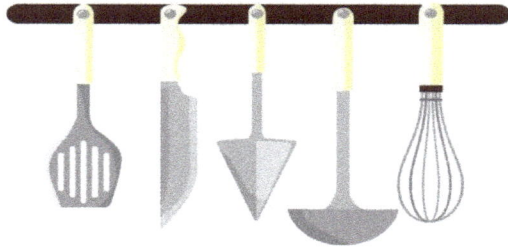

WHOLEMEAL TOZZETTI WITH HAZELNUT SEEDS AND CEREALS

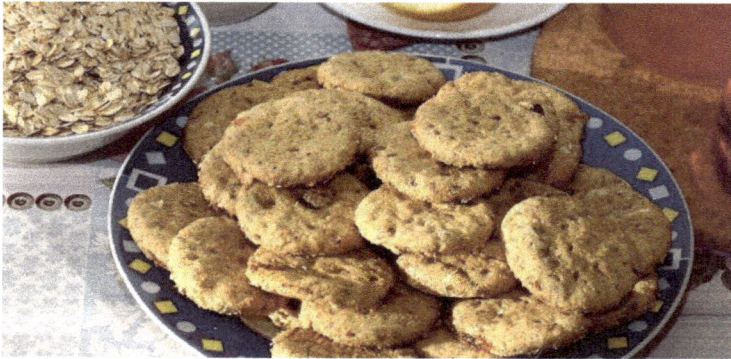

Times:

Preparation 10 min

Cooking 20 min

Roasting 4/5 min

Total 44/45 min

For 15 biscuits

For 1 biscuit / piece:

Nutritional values

Calories 84

Carbohydrates 7 gr

Fats 5 gr

Protein 3 gr

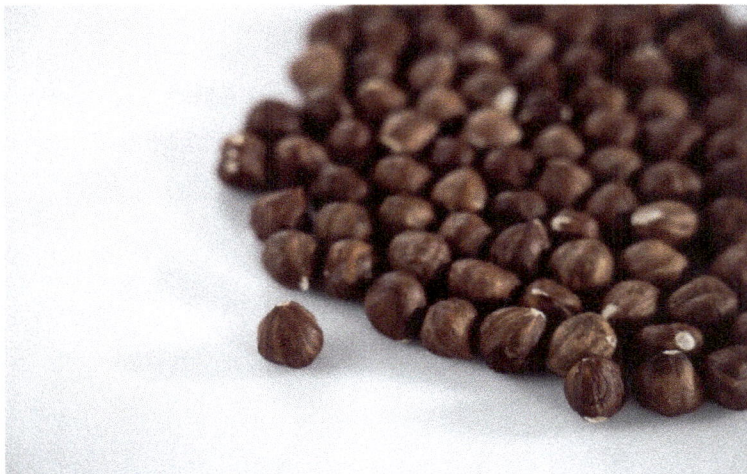

MATERIALS

1 baking sheet

1 bowl

INGREDIENTS

140 gr Flour with cereals and seeds

or whole meal

100 gr Erythritol or 80 gr Stevia

1 egg

1 Album

½ Teaspoon Yeast for cakes or bicarbonate

Zest of ½ lemon

Zest of ½ Orange

1 Pinch Salt

Cinnamon

100 gr Hazelnuts in grains or other dried fruit

INSTRUCTIONS

Preheat the oven to 170 ° degrees in ventilated mode for about 10 minutes, combine all the ingredients in a bowl and knead them well, kneading with your hands, until you get a pastry-like consistency. Now create a cylinder, working it on a surface or on the kitchen table, sprinkle with a pinch of powdered sweetener and bake for 20 minutes, cook until the surface of the dough is golden. Always useful to check the cooking with a toothpick if it was ready, remove it from the oven and slice it while it is still hot, bake again for toasting at 180 degrees, for 4 or 5 minutes per side.

Serve warm accompanied by a fragrant tea or herbal tea.

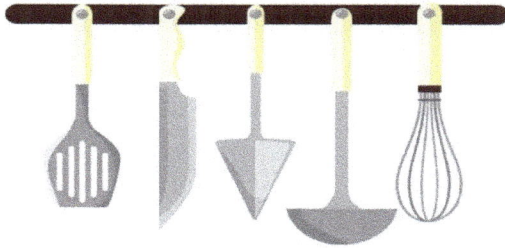

CHEESECAKE RASPBERRIES, BLUEBERRIES AND LEMON

This is a medium difficulty recipe for cooking a tasty cheesecake perfect for the ketogenic diet, this version of cheesecake has a very low carbohydrate dose compared to the original recipe and for this reason it is suitable for the Keto diet, but also for those who do not want they want to eat healthy, while not following a low-calorie diet.

It is also perfect for lactose intolerant, as it involves the use of lactose-free butter and cream cheese, and for celiacs thanks to the hazelnut flour. The latter contains fewer carbohydrates than the traditional one, and the biscuit placed at the base of this cake is gluten-free.

Basically, our Keto cheesecake is a greedy solution for many or perhaps everyone.

It is easily digestible and tasty, nutritious and energetic.

Times:

Preparation 20 min

Cooling down 30 min

Cooking 45 min

Total 1 hour and 35 min

For 6 people

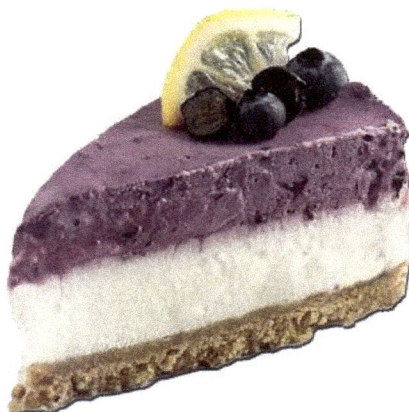

For 1 slice:

Nutritional values

Calories 375

Carbohydrates 11.9 gr

Fats 22.3 gr

Protein 8.8 gr

Fiber 4.4 gr

MATERIALS

Electric whips

1 hinged cake pan with a diameter of 20/22 cm

1 small saucepan

1 Spatula

2 Bowls

INGREDIENTS

For the base:

150 grams of hazelnut flour,

155 gr of chopped hazelnuts,

160 gr of clarified butter,

50 gr of Stevia (replace about 90/100 g of sugar)

For the cream:

750 gr of Lactose Free Creamy Cheese

6 eggs

Juice from 3 lemons

90 gr of Stevia (replace about 180 g of sugar)

For the decoration:

lime zest

raspberries

blueberries

INSTRUCTIONS

Put the butter in a saucepan and let it melt over low heat.
Put the flour and chopped hazelnuts in a bowl, add the melted
butter and Stevia, mix with a spatula to mix all the ingredients
together.
Use the mixture to coat the bottom and edges of a 20/22 cm
diameter springform pan.

Refrigerate for about 30 minutes, in order to harden the mixture, which serves as a base for your cheesecake.

Put the lactose-free cream cheese in another bowl and add the Stevia, the eggs and the juice of 3 lemons, mix all the ingredients well, this time using the electric whisk, until the mixture is smooth and homogeneous.

Remove the pan from the fridge and pour the cream on the hazelnut base, level the cream gently with a spoon over the entire surface.

Bake the cheesecake in the preheated oven at 175 degrees for about 40/45 minutes.

Remove from the oven and let it cool.

Decorate the cheesecake by distributing fresh raspberries and blueberries on the surface and finish with lime zest.

Serve it fresh and keep it in the fridge.

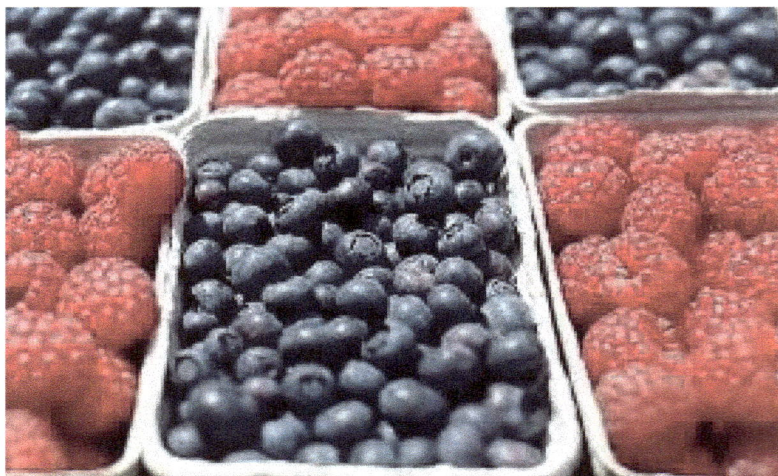

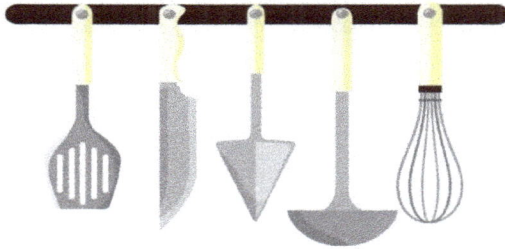

BUCKWHEAT BISCUIT SLICES

This recipe for rusks indicated for those who follow a ketogenic diet, is simple, but it must be followed step by step to obtain an alternative to the classic slices, but strictly sugar-free and gluten-free.

SUGAR FREE

GTUTEN FREE

Times:

Preparation 20 min

Cooking 40 min

Cooling and toasting 2 h 30 min

Total 3 h 30 min

For 25/26 slices

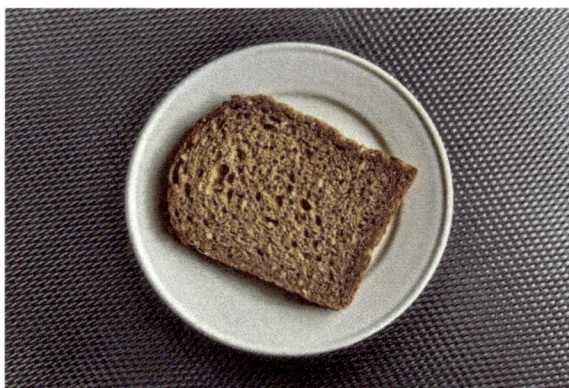

For 1 slice:

Nutritional values

Calories 55

Carbohydrates 5.19 gr

Ratio 2.39 gr

Fat 10.2 gr

Protein 3.73 gr

MATERIALS

Electric whips

1 Mold for plumcake 24 X 14 cm

3 Bowls

Greaseproof paper

INGREDIENTS

300 gr buckwheat or corn flour
(you can also combine them)

2 eggs

60 gr Erythritol or 30 gr of Stevia

200 ml of water

50 ml EVO oil or seed oil or coconut oil

2 gr salt

4 gr cream of tartar or baking powder

1/2 tsp baking soda

spices to taste... for example cinnamon

INSTRUCTIONS

Preheat the oven to 180 ° degrees preferably ventilated for 10 minutes, meanwhile in a bowl add the salt, baking soda, baking powder, spices and flour. In another bowl separate the yolks from the whites and whisk the egg whites until stiff peaks, preferably with medium speed electric whisk. Add the chosen sweetener to the egg yolks and whip the yolks as well until you get a com light and frothy place, add the chosen oil to the yolks and continue to mix, always at medium speed, now also add the water to the mixture of yolks and mix well. Now also add the flour with yeast and spices to the egg yolk mixture, then gently add the egg whites, whipping from bottom to top. The dough must be smooth, homogeneous and not to liquid, pour it into the loaf pan lined with parchment paper or greased or greased, and bake in the oven for 40 minutes, until golden brown. Gently remove it from the mold and let it cool completely. Cut the pancake into slices about ½ cm thick, obviously the thickness will depend on your tastes. To finish, proceed to the biscuit, preheating the oven to 160 ° degrees and cook for another 12/15 minutes per side.

Eat them warm or cold.

The slices keep for about 15 days in an airtight container.

Note:

The rusks can be flavored to taste, using your favorite spices, perfect with cinnamon, or nutmeg and cloves.

You can add raisins to the dough or dried fruit or chocolate chips, to make the slices even more delicious.

A second way to flavor them is to replace part of the water with another liquid, for example limoncello or marsala.

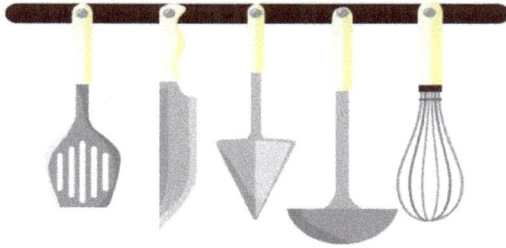

RICOTTA CAKE AND RED FRUITS

Times:

Preparation 10 min

Cooking 40 min

Total 50 min

For 8 people

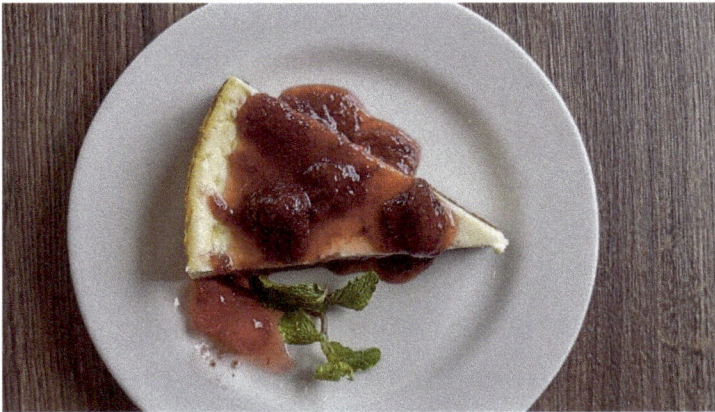

For 1 slice:

Nutritional values

Calories 110

Carbohydrates 5.5 gr

Sugars 6 gr

Fat 8 gr

Protein 4.5 gr

MATERIALS

Electric or hand whips

1 cake pan 16 cm

1 bowl

Greaseproof paper

INGREDIENTS

35 gr coconut flour

100 gr almond flour

120 ml vegetable milk or soy

90 gr lean ricotta

180 gr of egg whites

zest of 1 untreated lemon or lemon flavoring

½ sachet of baking powder or 1 teaspoon and ½ bicarbonate +
lemon juice

100 gr red fruits also frozen

120 gr Erythritol or 40 gr Stevia

INSTRUCTIONS

Preheat the oven in preferably ventilated mode, at 180 ° degrees
for about 10 minutes, add the flours together with the yeast,
mix carefully and slowly, so that they are then distributed
evenly in the dough.

Combine the egg white and ricotta together, lightly whipping the mixture, also add the sweetener of your choice and the lemon zest or the aroma, continuing to mix until it is completely dissolved and you have obtained a frothy mixture. At this point, add the flours a little at a time and continue mixing.

You will notice that the mixture is very solid, add the milk a little at a time until you get a consistency of the right density.

Gently incorporate the red fruits into the mixture and pour everything into the pan lined with parchment paper, now cook for about 40 minutes always at 180 degrees.

Test the toothpick before baking!

Serve lukewarm.

Note:

I advise you to decorate with special icing sugar, blend 100 g of Erythritol with 10 g of corn starch or 40 g of Stevia with 4 g of starch.

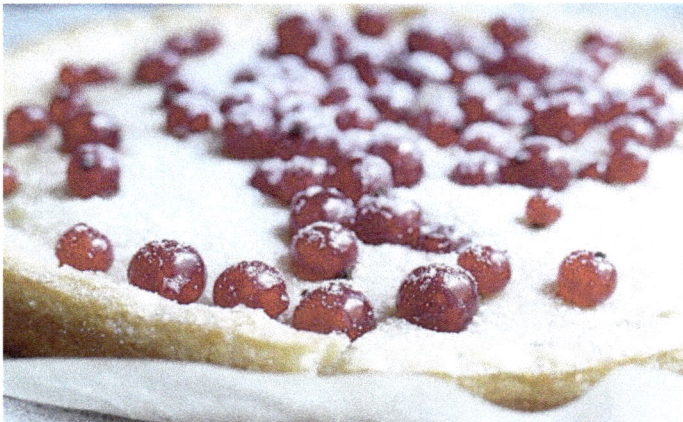

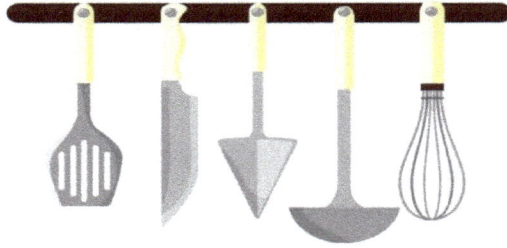

COCONUT CREAM

Quick and easy recipe to make, perfect for filling sweets and cakes in a healthy way.

Low-carb, ketogenic.

Ready in 5 minutes.

Times:

Preparation 5 min

Cooking 5 min

Total 10 min

For 200 gr of cream

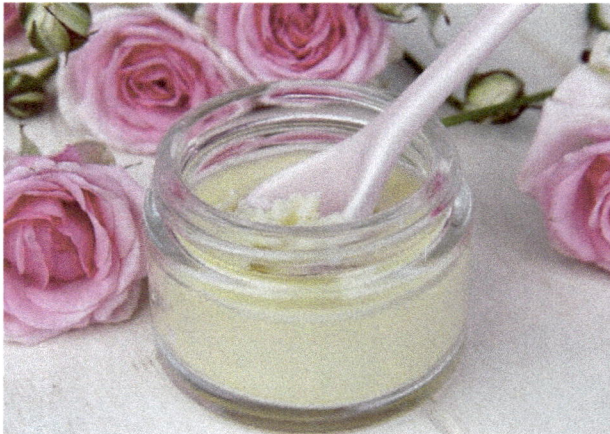

For 100 gr:

Nutritional values

Calories 130

Carbohydrates 3.5 gr

Sugars 2 gr

Fats 10.5 gr

Protein 6 gr

MATERIALS

Electric whips

1 small saucepan

INGREDIENTS

100 gr canned coconut milk

100 gr egg white

5 gr de-fat coconut flour

5 gr rapé coconut

10 drops coconut flavdrops

(or favorite sweetener)

INSTRUCTIONS

In a saucepan, combine all the ingredients, then put it over medium / low heat, making sure to turn and stir often, when it becomes thick, remove it from the heat and let it cool. Then blend it with an electric whisk and use it as you prefer, to fill sweets or by itself with a spoon.

Keep it in the fridge.

Note:

Canned coconut milk is thick and high in good fats, if you substitute with a coconut drink you will need more coconut flour to thicken.

You can replace the flavdrops with your favorite sweetener to taste. or 1 tablespoon of Erythritol.

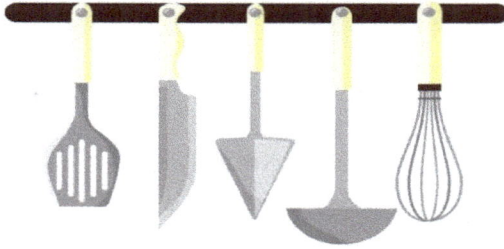

FERRERO ROCHER LIGHT

Particularly simple recipe and without cooking.

These Ferrero Rocher Ketogenic chocolates are sugar-free, have a creamy, melt-in-your-mouth heart and are coated in crunchy, dark chocolate.

Times:

Preparation 10 min

Total 10 min

Servings 10 chocolates

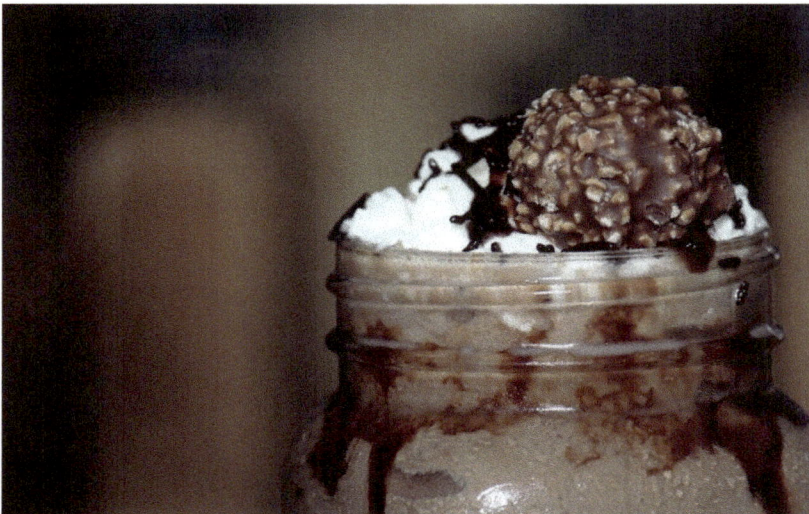

For 1 chocolate:

Nutritional values

Calories 90

Carbohydrates 2.5 gr

Sugars 1 gr

Protein 4 g r

Fat 7 gr

MATERIALS

1 small saucepan

1 small bowl

1 saucer

INGREDIENTS

30 gr unsweetened cocoa powder

20 gr butter

20 gr chocolate proteins

20 gr unsweetened almond milk (or preferred)

9 hazelnuts

q.s. peanuts

q.s. 85% dark chocolate

INSTRUCTIONS

Melt the butter in a saucepan over low heat, add the cocoa, proteins and milk, turn and mix carefully, now divide this dough into 9 portions of about 10 gr, divide each portion into two parts and with the 2 formed parts two circles, put 1 hazelnut on a circle and cover with the other circle, working it with your hands, continue like this also with the other 8 parts of the dough.

Work all 9 parts into balls.

Put some water in a small bowl and the chopped peanuts in a saucer. pass the balls in the water quickly and then pass them in the saucer with the chopped peanuts. Continue like this until all the balls are covered. Now melt the dark chocolate over low heat or in the microwave or in a double boiler. With the help of 2 forks, pass one ball at a time in the melted chocolate, so for all the others. Cover all the balls and let the chocolate harden, better by putting them in the fridge or freezer.

Ready, healthy and super greedy!

Perfect as a snack and an immediate source of energy. Store in the fridge.

Note:

You can use either butter or coconut oil, the former obviously contains lactose but has fewer calories than the latter.

Proteins are used to give more taste and sweetness, you can replace them with the same weight of another dry ingredient.

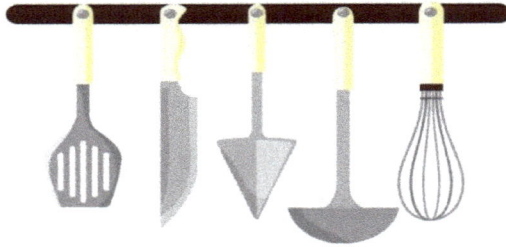

MINICAKE CREAM AND ALMONDS

This recipe is very simple and quick and you only need 5 ingredients and a bowl to prepare a snack, a breakfast or a greedy snack, within a Keto diet, without sugar and gluten.

Times:

Preparation 10 min

Cooking 20 min

Total 30 min

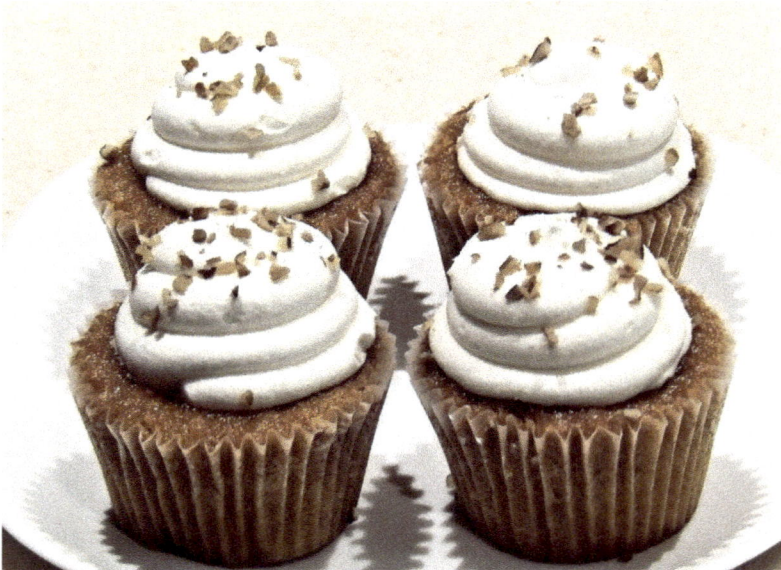

For 1 pie:

Nutritional values

Calories 330

Carbohydrates 5 gr

Sugars 2.5 gr

Protein 11 gr

Fat 29.5 gr

MATERIALS

1 bowl

1 Mold with a diameter of about 10/12 cm

INGREDIENTS

1 egg

50 gr fresh cream

20 gr almond flour

5 gr psyllium cuticles powder

1 tablespoon erythritol

1 pinch baking powder

(or cream of tartar or baking soda)

q.s. vanilla

INSTRUCTIONS

For this recipe, preheat the oven to 180 degrees for about 10 minutes, you can also cook the pie in the microwave or steam.

Break the egg into a bowl, add the cream and a pinch of salt and beat lightly with a fork.

Add all the other ingredients, mix carefully, making sure to combine them evenly.

Pour into the chosen mold and cook for about 15/20 minutes.

Let cool, cut horizontally and stuffed to taste with fantasy.

Note:

You can replace the almond flour with others you prefer and use,

You can replace Erythritol with another sweetener, I prefer it as it is very similar to sugar but has 0 calories, low glycemic index and is natural.

You can replace fresh cream with Greek yogurt, thus lowering the calories as well.

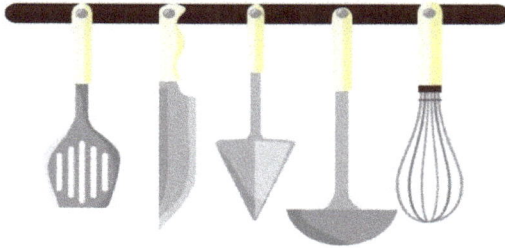

SOFT LIGHT NOUGAT

Soft Nougat Light prepared with only 3 main ingredients and very quick to prepare, very good and without sugar, perfect for everyone, in any diet and very low-calorie.

Times:

Preparation 15 min

Freezing 60 min

Total time 1 hour and 15 min

For 8 bars

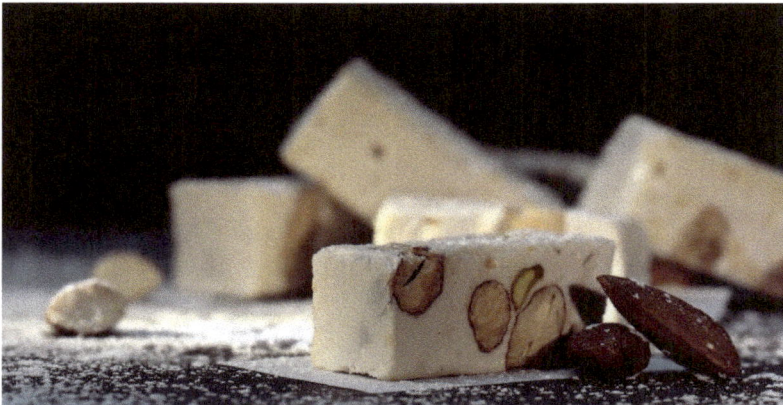

For 1 bar:

Nutritional values

Calories 65

Carbohydrates 3 gr

Sugars 1.5 gr

Protein 3 gr

Fats 4.5 gr

MATERIALS

Electric whips

1 Silicone mold

1 small saucepan

1 bowl

INGREDIENTS

For the Nougat:

50 gr almond flour

1 egg

30 gr Erythritol

10 gr Degreased coconut flour

q.s. vanilla and lemon zest

For the Caramel (optional):

15 gr 100% peanut butter

10 gr maple syrup

q.s. unsweetened vegetable milk

INSTRUCTIONS

Put the erythritol in a saucepan with about 20 grams of water and melt over low heat, when it is dissolved add all the other ingredients and keep the heat low, until everything thickens.

Pour the mixture into a silicone mold, of any shape and place in the freezer for 30 minutes.

Now add the peanut butter to the maple syrup and add the milk slowly until you get a thick caramel.

Pour over the cold nougat, spread and put back in the freezer for another 30 minutes.

Cut into bars and eat, the rest will keep in the fridge.

Note:

You can also make almond flour yourself at home, by blending the peeled almonds.

You could also substitute peanut butter with other nut butter. For the ketogenic diet, on the other hand, you can omit the maple syrup, diluting the peanut butter with milk only and adding a teaspoon of Erythritol.

Erythritol is very similar in flavor to sugar but has 0 calories, low glycemic
index, is natural and has no unpleasant aftertaste.

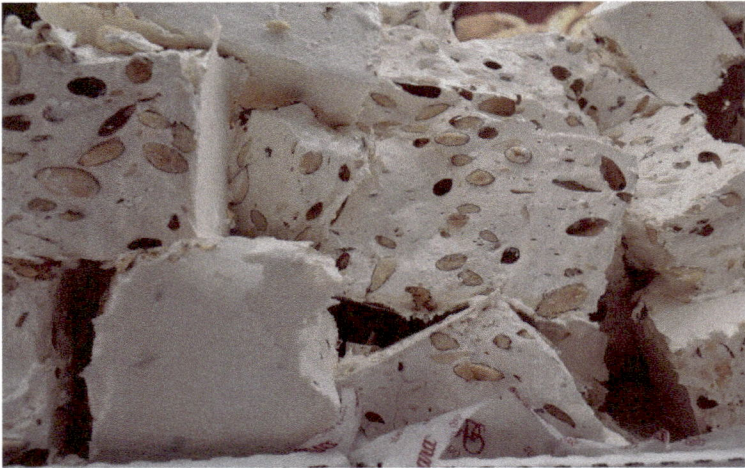

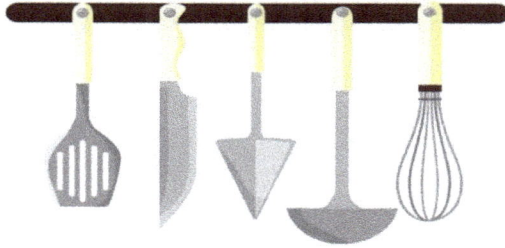

PEANUT BUTTER PROTEIN CREAM

This recipe will serve you to make a peanut butter protein cream of exceptional density with only 3 ingredients, very fast and low-calorie.

Times:

Preparation 5minutes

Cooking 5 minutes

Total 10 min

For 2 people (220 gr of cream)

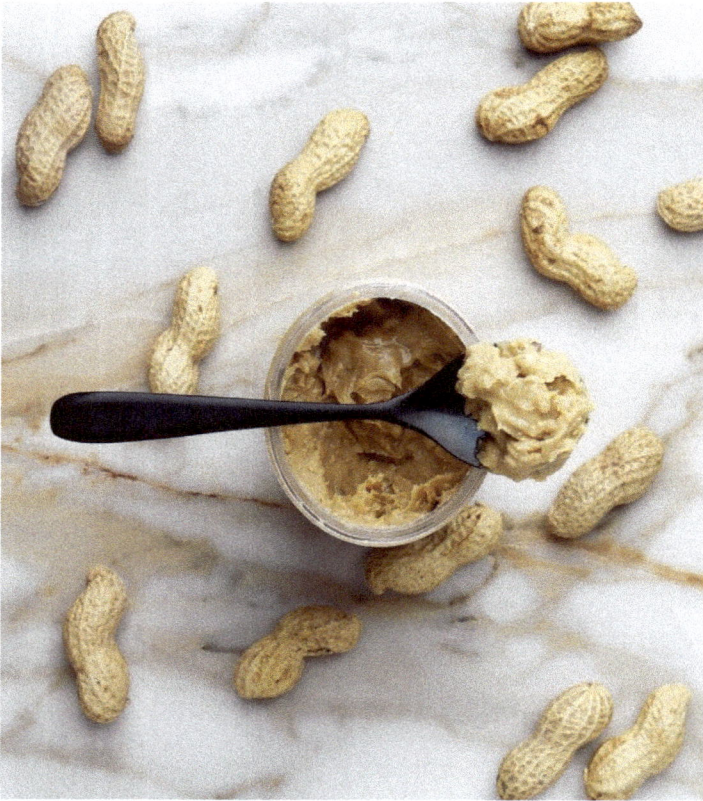

For 1 person (110 gr):

Nutritional values

Calories 110

Carbohydrates 3.5 gr

Sugars 2 gr

Protein 11 gr

Fat 6 gr

MATERIALS

Mixer

1 small saucepan

INGREDIENTS

100 gr egg white

100 gr unsweetened vegetable milk

20 gr 100% peanut butter

20 gr powdered peanut butter

2 tablespoons Erythritol

1/2 teaspoon of cinnamon

INSTRUCTION

Combine all the ingredients in a saucepan and mix everything over a low heat, when it is thickened, turn off and let it cool.

Blend and then place in the fridge.

You can use the cream in many ways, to fill a cake, spread on bread or on its own with a spoon.

It can be kept in the fridge for 2/3 days.

Note:

You can replace the powdered peanut butter with a starch, but lose a little in flavor.

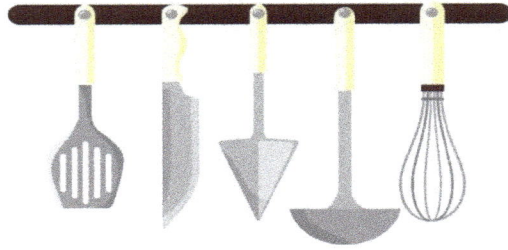

DARK COCOA CAKE

Cocoa fondant cake is an amazingly good and equally easy-to-make, healthy, gluten-free, low-carb and keto-free cake.

Times:

Preparation 10 min

Cooking 15 min

Total 25 min

For 6 people

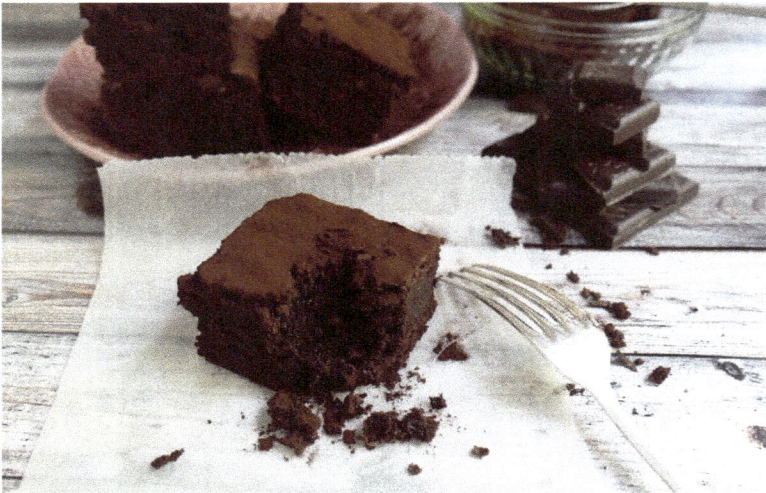

For 1 slice of cake without topping:

Nutritional values

Calories 250

Carbohydrates 7 gr

Sugars 4 gr

Protein 13.5 gr

Fats 18.5 gr

MATERIALS

Electric or hand whips

1 silicone cake pan with a diameter of about 20 cm

1 bowl

INGREDIENTS

1 egg

50 gr thick coconut milk

10 gr Cocoa

5 gr almond flour

5 gr de-fat coconut flour

5 gr powdered peanut butter *

1 pinch of baking powder

q.s. Vanilla flavor

1 tablespoon erythritol

Peanut Butter Powder allows you to

have the same taste but with fewer calories.

INSTRUCTIONS

Preheat the oven to 180 degrees for about 10 minutes.

Break the egg into a bowl, add the coconut milk, vanilla and a pinch of salt and whip by hand with a fork or with an electric mixer at low speed.

add all the other ingredients and mix carefully making the mixture homogeneous.

Pour the mixture into a 20 cm mold in the oven for about 15 minutes, or you can use muffin cups or you could cook the cake in a cup in the microwave for 4/5 minutes.

You can add the topping, to make it even tastier, using 10 g of Chocolate Protein Cream, diluted with a drop of almond milk.

Note:

You can replace Coconut Milk with Greek Yogurt.

Erythritol is, as you know, a 100% Natural sweetener without aftertaste, very similar to Sugar and with 0 calories, but you can replace it with another sweetener, remembering that it could change the consistency of the dough.

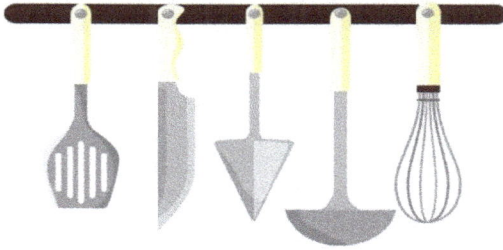

PANETTONE

This recipe will serve you to make a very famous Christmas dessert in a keto, low-carb and gluten-free version.

Follow all the steps carefully and carefully.

Times:

Preparation 15 min

Rising 8 hours

Cooking 40 min

Total time 8 hours and 55 mins min

For 1 Panettone of about 500 gr

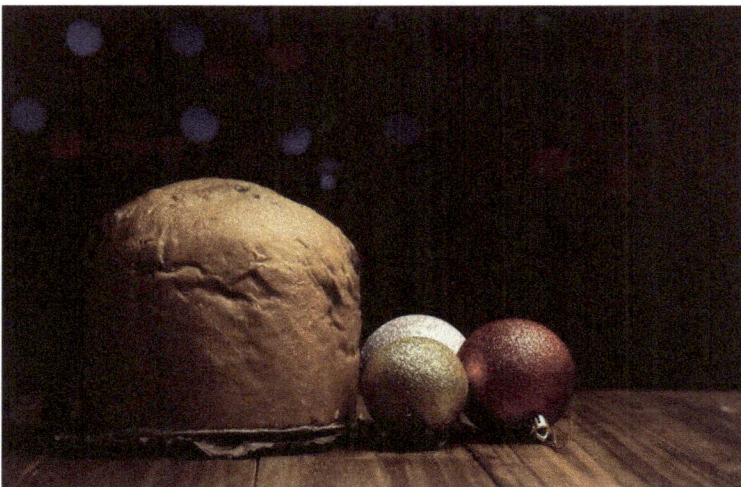

For 1 slice of Panettone:

Nutritional values

Calories 201

Carbohydrates 1.4 gr

Ratio 2.71 gr

Protein 13.5 gr

Fat 1.78 gr

Protein 5.21 gr

MATERIALS

Electric whips

1 High mold specific for panettone

1 bowl

1 Strainer

1 small saucepan

INGREDIENTS

280 gr Ketomix flour pan

70 gr Erythritol

2 eggs

50 gr Butter

8 gr Fresh brewer's yeast

80 gr Almond milk

50 gr 90% dark chocolate

10 drops of dietic

10 almonds to decorate

INSTRUCTIONS

Sift the flour with a tightly meshed sieve to remove all the seeds, add the erythritol and the eggs, mix and knead, dissolve the yeast in the almond milk in a saucepan over low heat and add it to the previous mixture, continuing to mix, now instead use low speed electric whips.

Add the butter at room temperature and the chocolate into small pieces, add the dietetic sweetener and place everything in a 500 kg panettone mold.

Decorate with almonds and leave to rise in the oven off, but with the light on for at least 8 hours.

Bake in a static oven at 180 degrees for 40 minutes.

Serve warm or cold.

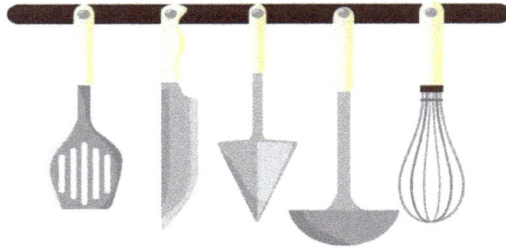

DRIED FRUIT BARS

Dried fruit bars are really easy to prepare at home, ideal for breakfast or a snack, but also as a mid-morning snack they are great.

Times:

Preparation 10 min

Cooking 10 min

Total 20 min

For 8 bars

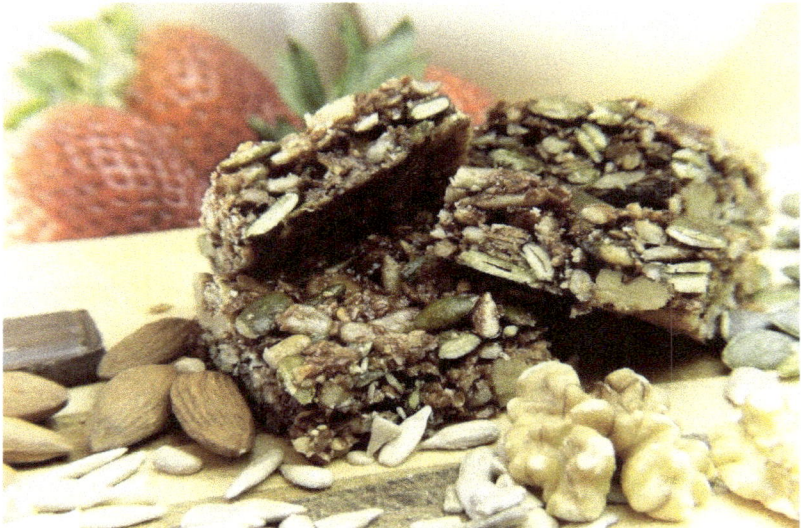

For 1 bar:

Nutritional values

Calories 154

Carbohydrates 1.50 gr

Ratio 1.82 gr

Fat 1.34 gr

Protein 5.86 gr

MATERIALS

Electric or hand whips

1 Rectangular baking mold about 30x10 cm

Greaseproof paper

INGREDIENTS

130 gr hazelnuts

30 gr chopped pistachios

70 gr pumpkin seeds

2 egg whites

20 gr of Erythritol

INSTRUCTIONS

For this recipe, cut the hazelnuts coarsely and add them to the chopped pistachios, pumpkin seeds, egg whites and Erythritol, mix and mix everything well with electric whisk triche or hand and place the mixture in a rectangular mold of about 30 x 10 cm, with parchment paper.

Now cook in a ventilated oven at 200 ° degrees for 10 minutes. Let it cool, then cut it into slices and, if you prefer, also into smaller pieces to use as a snack.

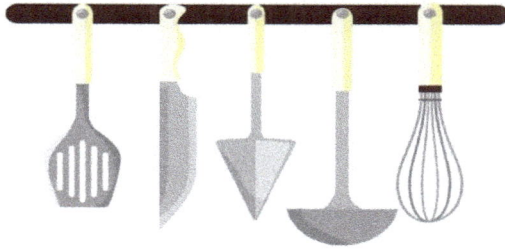

TRUFFLE HAZELNUTS

Recipe for children, healthy and delicious.

Snack with energy in a few calories!

Times:

Preparation 15 min

Total 15 min

For 4/6 people

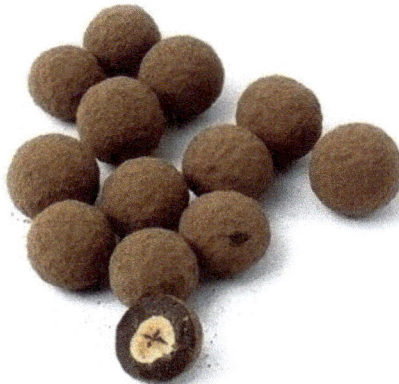

For 1 hazelnut:

Nutritional values

Calories 75

Carbohydrates 1.05 gr

Ratio 2.28 gr

Fats 6.67 gr

Protein 1.98 gr

MATERIALS

1 non-stick pan

1 bowl

1 Strainer

INGREDIENTS

100 gr peeled hazelnuts

100 gr erythritol

30 gr butter

20 gr unsweetened cocoa powder

INSTRUCTIONS

To prepare the truffled hazelnuts, start by putting the cocoa in a bowl, while at the same time putting the erythritol and the butter in a non-stick pan, melt both until the erythritol becomes liquid.

Remove the pan from the heat and add the hazelnuts, stirring.

Take the bowl with the cocoa and put the hazelnuts a little at a time and with the help of a teaspoon round them a little and cover them with cocoa, hurry up because the erythritol cools quickly.

Let the hazelnuts cool and pass them in a tightly meshed colander to remove the excess cocoa.

Ready to be eaten, perfect at any time of the day.

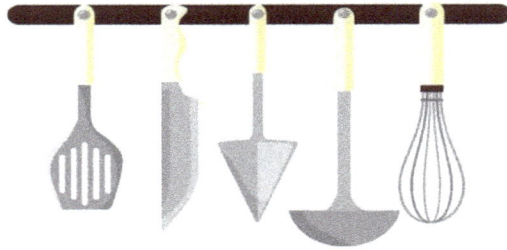

COCONUT BISCUITS

This biscuit recipe is perfect in a ketogenic diet, that is a diet with very low carbohydrates content, but with proteins and high in fat.

They are low in sugar, but at the same time very caloric, it is advisable to consume 20/30 grams per day.

Times:

Preparation 10 min

Freezing 3 hours

Total 3 hours and 10 min

For about 20 biscuits

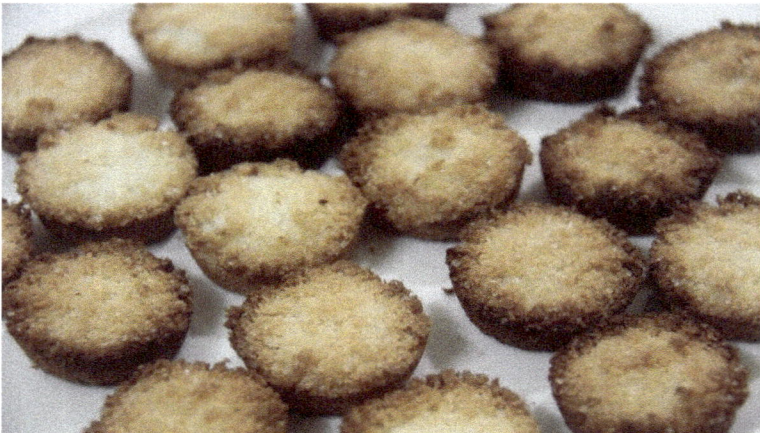

For 30 grams of biscuits:

Nutritional values

Calories 138

Carbohydrates 0.3 gr

Fat 12.8 gr

Protein 3.7 gr

MATERIALS

Electric or hand whips

INGREDIENTS

100 gr Coconut flour

4 tablespoons of coconut oil

2 sachets of sweetener

INSTRUCTIONS

This coconut cookie recipe is super easy and quick, in fact you just need to mix all the ingredients.

Then you will have to form balls or the typical shape of the biscuit or at your pleasure different shapes and put them in the freezer for at least 3 hours.

After 3 hours they will be ready to be served.

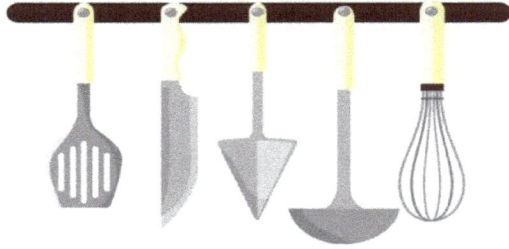

PANDORO

Keto, gluten-free and low-carb version of the famous Christmas dessert.

Times:

Preparation 10 min

Cooking 60 min

Total 1 hour and 10 min

For 6/8 people

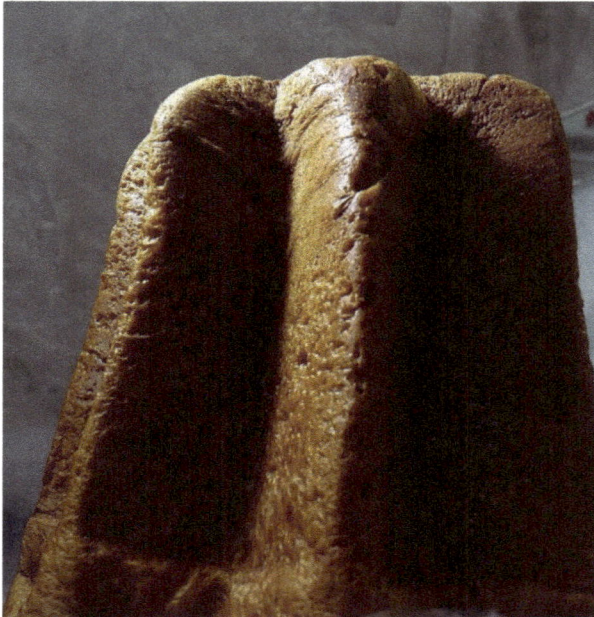

For 1 slice:

Nutritional values

Calories 208

Carbohydrates 6 gr

Fiber 2.8 gr

Fat 19.4 gr

Protein 5.8 gr

MATERIALS

Electric whips

1 mold for pandoro

INGREDIENTS

150 grams of almond flour

100 gr of icing erythritol

20 grams of coconut flour

20 gr of bamboo fiber

3 eggs

70 ml of melted butter

1/2 sachet of vanilla yeast

100 ml of coconut or regular cream

1 teaspoon of xanthan gum

vanilla flavor

INSTRUCTIONS

This recipe is the keto variant of the famous Christmas cake, to start preparing it, mix all the dry ingredients, add the eggs and cream and continue to mix vigorously and carefully, by hand or with electric whisk, paying particular attention to eliminate any lumps.

Now put the dough in a pandoro mold and bake
in static mode at 180 degrees for 1 hour.
Let it cool and decorate with icing erythritol.
Serve!

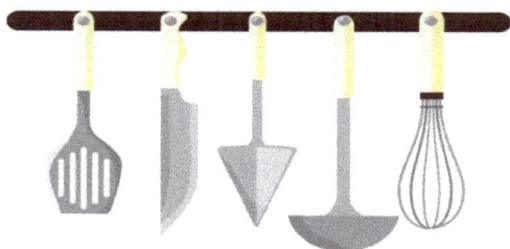

CHOCOLATE WITH DRIED FRUITS

Quick recipe for 16 chocolate squares to garnish
with what you prefer.

Super delicious snack!

Times:

Preparation 10 min

Cooling down 30 min

Total 40 min

For 16 pieces / squares

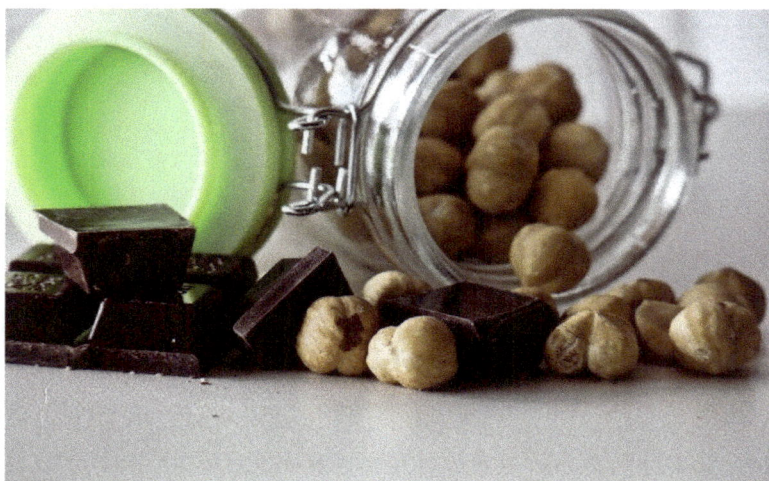

For 1 piece:

Nutritional values

Calories 147

Carbohydrates 1.92 gr

Ratio 2.35 gr

Fat 1.24 gr

Protein 3.33 gr

MATERIALS

2 rectangular containers of disposable
aluminum 13x10 cm approximately
1 small saucepan
1 Cylindrical container or large glass

INGREDIENTS

200 gr 99% dark chocolate
15 gr chopped pistachios
30 gr hazelnuts

INSTRUCTIONS

This recipe is very simple and quick, cut the hazelnuts coarsely
and put them on one side, they will be used to mitigate the too
bitter taste of the chocolate.

Melt the chocolate in the microwave and divide it into two
rectangular containers 13x10 cm, if they are more comfortable

for you you can also use 2 disposable aluminum trays, more or less of the same size.

Sprinkle the chopped pistachios in a bowl over the melted chocolate and cover the chocolate with the chopped hazelnuts in the other bowl.

Put in the freezer for at least 30 minutes.

Cut into 16 squares and serve the 2 different flavors if you like with a little sugar-free whipped cream next to them.

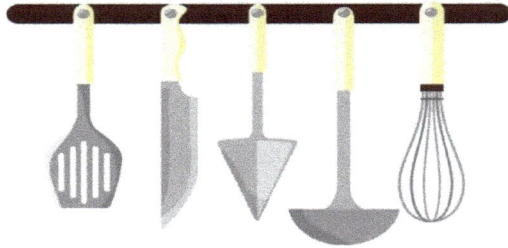

MASCARPONE CAKE WITH COCOA AND RUM

This is a sister recipe of the better known Tiramisu, equally
greedy here in a low-carb, gluten-free
and absolutely ketogenic version.

GLUTEN FREE

Times:

Preparation 20 min

Cooking 10 min

Cooling 3 hours

Total 3 hours and 30 min

For 6/8 people

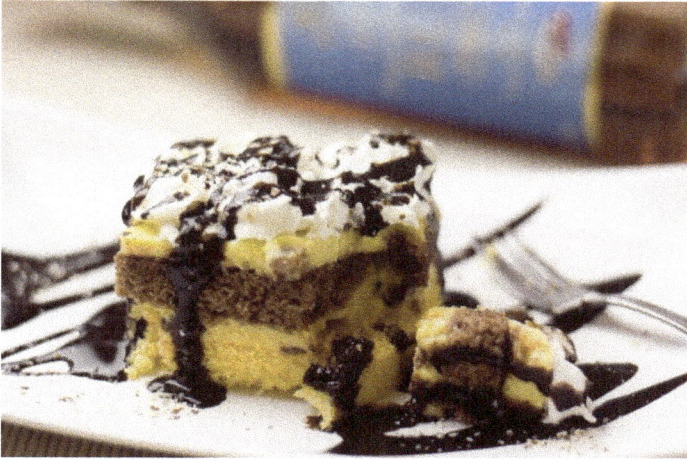

For 1 person:

Nutritional values

Calories 250

Carbohydrates 2 gr

Sugars 1.5 gr

Fat 19.5 gr

Protein 4 gr

MATERIALS

Electric whips

2 Bowls

1 rectangular cake pan

Greaseproof paper

INGREDIENTS

8 tablespoons of stevia powder (or 1 liquid)

2 Cups of almond flour

1 tablespoon of unsweetened cocoa

2 Spoons of coconut flour

120 gr of butter

240 gr of spreadable cheese (or ricotta)

1 cup of cream for desserts

300 grams of mascarpone

rum flavoring

1 sachet of vanillin

1 cup of coffee with sweetener

INSTRUCTIONS

For the mascarpone, cocoa and rum cake, mix the almond flour, coconut flour, 5 tablespoons of stevia, melted butter and vanilla in a bowl.

Mix the dough well and roll it out on a sheet of baking paper, cut it into rectangles and bake at 180 degrees for about 10 minutes, bake anyway until the rectangles are golden.

Separately, whip the cream with the remaining sweetener, and in another bowl, first mix the mascarpone, spreadable cheese and vanillin, then add the previously whipped cream, until everything is well blended and fluid.

Put the previously prepared rectangles / biscuits in a rectangular pan and sprinkle them with coffee sweetened and flavored with a vial of rum flavoring.

Now add a layer of cream with mascarpone and cream and alternate another layer of biscuits and one of mascarpone cream.

Complete the cake with a sprinkling of cocoa.

Refrigerate for at least 3 hours before serving.

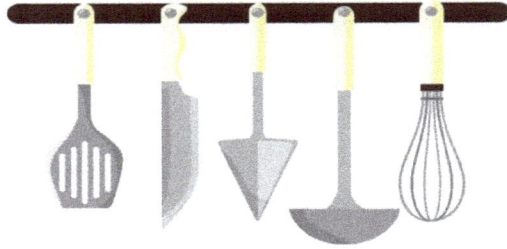

AVOCADO BROWNIE

This recipe is simple, fast and delicious, in addition, chocolate has a positive effect on mood and avocado contains a huge amount of potassium.

GLUTEN FREE

Times:

Preparation 10 min

Cooking 20/25 min

Total 35 min

For 6 people

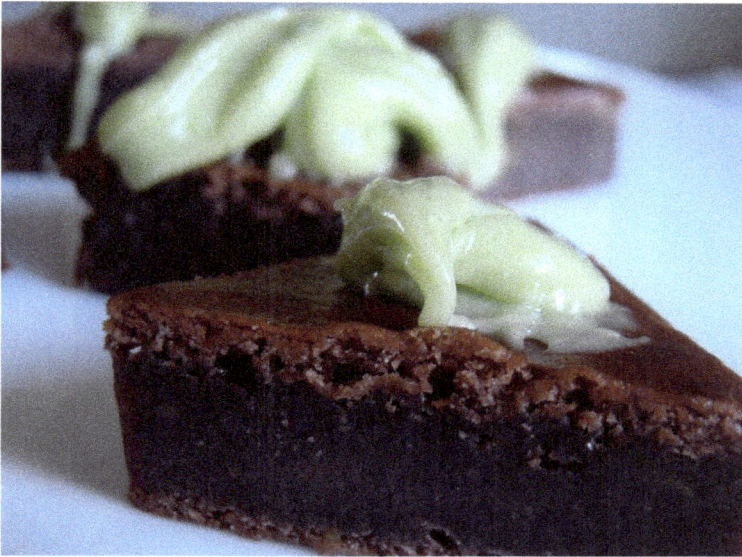

For 1 slice:

Nutritional values

Calories 183

Carbohydrates 4.9 gr

Fats 16.6 gr

Protein 1.4 gr

MATERIALS

Electric mixer or whisks

1 rectangular bowl

Greaseproof paper

INGREDIENTS

2 Avocado

4 eggs

6 Tbsp peanut butter (unsweetened)

3 cups of coconut flour

2 tablespoons of yeast

3 tablespoons of cocoa (unsweetened)

3 tablespoons of sweetener

4 tablespoons of butter

1 pinch of salt

vanilla extract

INSTRUCTIONS

Prepare all the ingredients and put them in a blender to blend until the dough is smooth, fluid and homogeneous.

Pour everything into a rectangular pan, with parchment paper on the bottom, and bake with ventilated mode, preferably at 180 degrees for about 20/25 min.

Try the toothpick and the brownies are ready!

Let cool and serve.

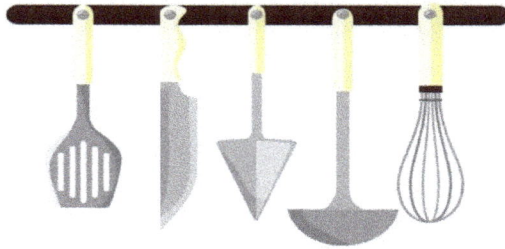

BUSTRENGO

In Romagna, an Italian region they cook a rustic sweet of breadcrumbs which is a poor recovery recipe, called bustrengo. There are many different recipes mixing old bread with fruit to make a homemade dessert or enriched only with pine nuts and raisins. After removing the raisins, which we will replace with blueberries, and obviously the sugar, half replaced by erythritol, here is the recipe for a ketogenic, easy and cheap bustrengo.

GLUTEN FREE

Times:

Preparation 10 min

Cooking 25 min

Total 35 min

For 6 people

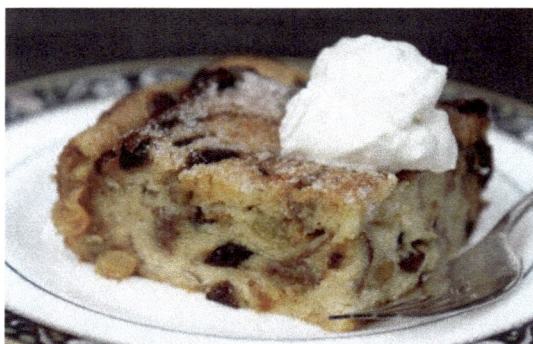

For 100 gr of dessert:

Nutritional values

Calories 189

Carbohydrates 14.85 gr

Ratio 1.36 gr

Fat 10.8 gr

Protein 36.54 gr

MATERIALS

Electric whips

1 Rectangular mold 10x17 cm

Greaseproof paper

INGREDIENTS

80 gr almond flour

30 gr rapé coconut

(or 110 gr only almond flour)

15 gr psyllium

165 gr whole milk

35 gr melted butter

30 gr egg (1/2 large egg)

0.5 gr anise seeds

0.4 gr cinnamon powder

1/2 lemon grated zest

0.07 gr sucralose

45 gr blueberries

15 gr pine nuts

INSTRUCTIONS

Mix all the ingredients, leaving only blueberries and pine nuts
on one side.

Pour into a 10 x 17 cm rectangular mold, usually the rectangular
shape is easily found, line it with baking paper, level the
mixture well.

Now put the blueberries on top of the surface of the dough and
finally the

Pine nuts.

Bake at 175 degrees for about 25 minutes.

Unlike other sweets, its characteristic is that it must remain
moist inside.

Serve lukewarm.

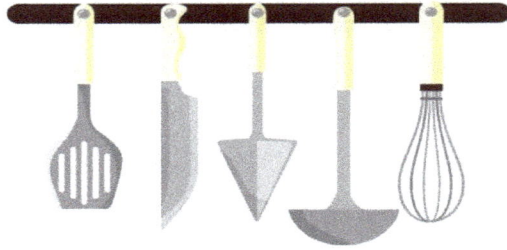

CHOCOLATE AND CHEESECAKE

Super delicious and healthy cake, respecting the rules of the keto diet, relax by making a cake of medium difficulty.

GLUTEN FREE

Times:

Preparation 20 min

Cooking 30 min

Total 50 min

For 6/8 people

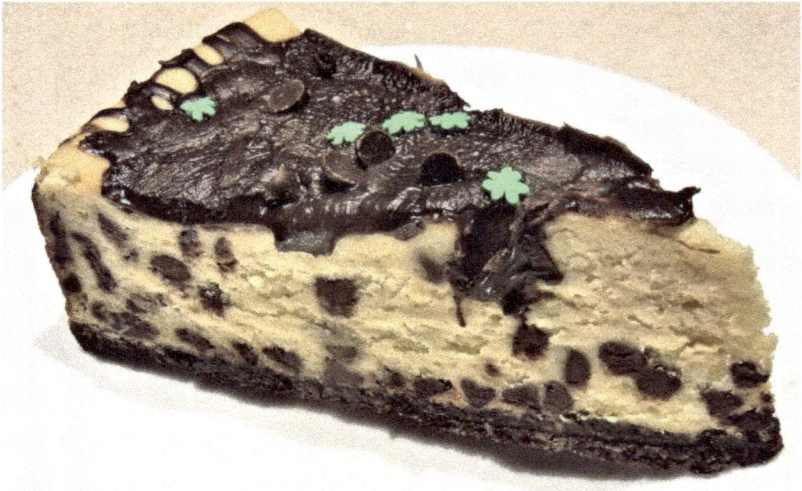

For 1 slice:

Nutritional values

Calories 140

Carbohydrates 1.7 gr

Sugars. 1.3 gr

Fat 11.5 gr

Proteins 6 gr

MATERIALS

Electric whips

Cake pan ofameter 20 cm

1 small saucepan

2 Bowls

INGREDIENTS

200 gr of cream cheese such
as Philadelphia

100 gr 90% dark chocolate

50 gr Erythritol

4 eggs

5 drops tic

Ketoneural protein fdl

INSTRUCTIONS

Whip the egg yolks with cream cheese like Philadelphia, tic and erythritol, melt the chocolate in a double boiler and add it to the previously whipped mixture, add the whipped egg whites.

Now put the mixture in a pan with a diameter of about 20 cm, lined with baking paper, or oiled or buttered on the bottom, fill the baking sheet with water and cook the cake in a bain-marie for 15 minutes in a static oven at 180 degrees , then lower to 170 degrees for another 15 minutes.

Let the cake cool in the switched off oven with the door slightly open.

Sprinkle the surface of the cake with the fdl proteins as soon as it has cooled down.

The cake is ready to eat warm.

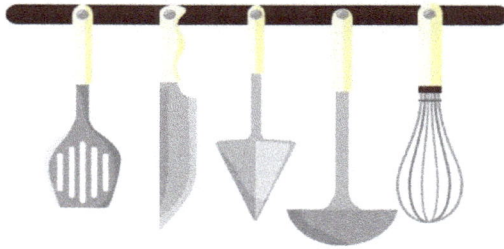

CINNAMON COOKIES

This recipe is quick and fun to make with the kids or on your

own to break the routine

on a boring afternoon.

GLUTEN FREE

Times:

Preparation 10 min

Cooking 15 minutes

Total 25 min

For 24 cookies

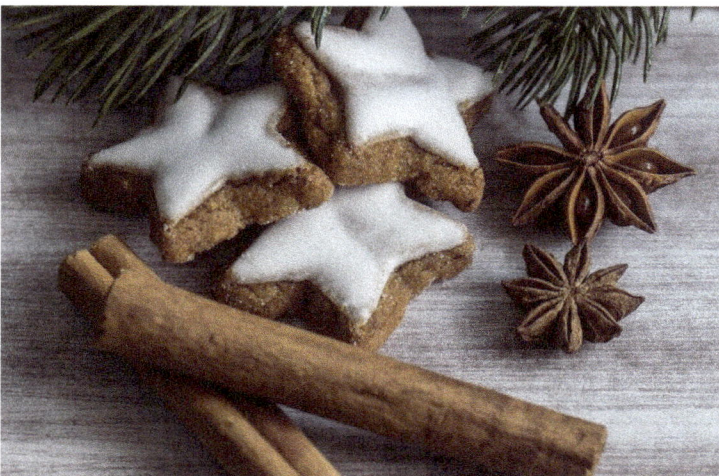

For 1 biscuit:

Nutritional values

Calories 41

Carbohydrates 7 gr

Sugars 1 gr

Fat 1 gr

Protein 1 gr

MATERIALS

Mixer or blender

1 Baking tray or baking tray

Greaseproof paper

INGREDIENTS

250 gr peeled almonds

50 gr erythritol

50 gr butter

1 egg

5 gr cinnamon powder

INSTRUCTIONS

Prepare all your tools and start by putting the almonds, erythritol and cinnamon in a blender or hand blender, chopping all the ingredients until they reach the consistency of flour.

Now add the egg, the butter into small pieces and continue to whisk.

After you have finished blending, gradually take the mixture and work it with your hands into 24 balls and place them gently on a baking sheet lined with baking paper.

Mash the balls giving them the round, classic shape of biscuits and finally bake in a convection oven at 180 degrees for 13/15 minutes.

Serve the cookies cold to appreciate their flavor more.

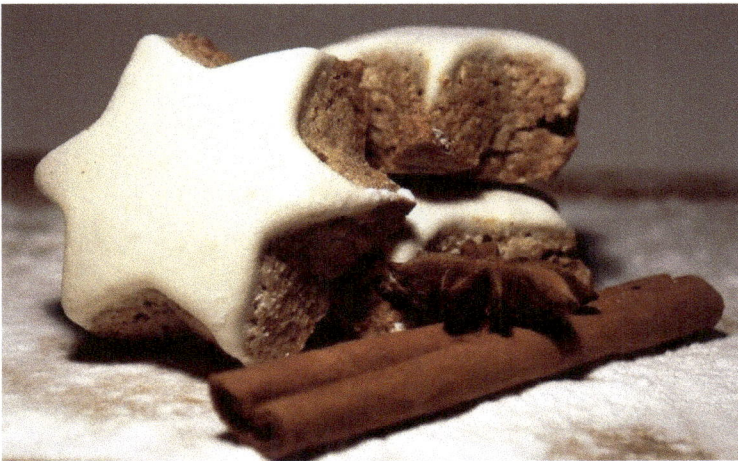

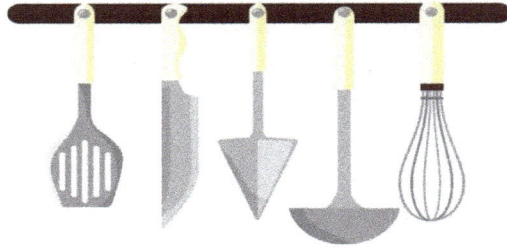

GINGER COOKIES

This recipe is quick and creative
for decorating your cookies.
Enjoy yourselves!
GLUTEN FREE

Times:

Preparation 20 min
Cooking 20/25 min
Total 40/45 min
For about 25 biscuits

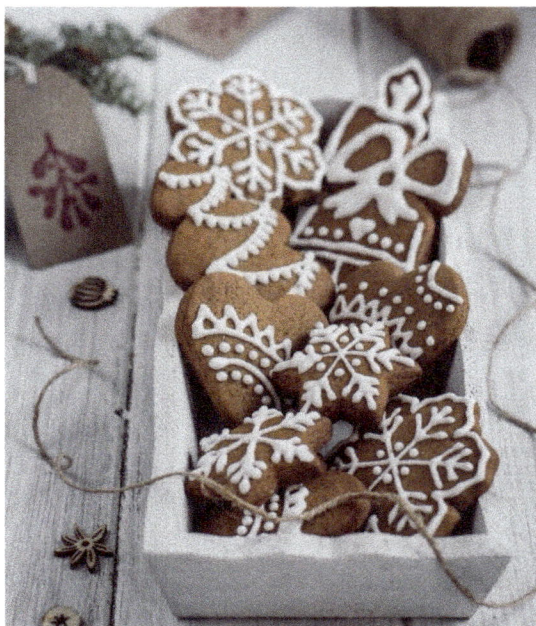

For 1 biscuit:

Nutritional values

Calories 67

Net carbohydrates 0.5 gr

Fats 16.45 gr

Protein 1.52 gr

MATERIALS

Planetary

1 Rolling pin

Electric whips

2 Bowls

1 baking sheet

Greaseproof paper

1 Sac a poche

For the dough

200 gr ketomix first courses

150 grams of almond flour

100 gr of erythriol

5 gr of powdered ginger

5 gr of cinnamon

A pinch of nutmeg

A pinch of cloves

1/2 teaspoon of baking soda

2 eggs

For the ice

1 egg white

100 gr of dietor powder

A few drops of lemon

INSTRUCTIONS

Put all the ingredients for the dough together, knead everything by hand or in a planetary mixer, roll out the dough and pull it until it reaches a layer of about 3/4 mm with a rolling pin and have fun giving it many different shapes by hand or with the molds, bake at 180 degrees for 20/25 minutes.

Whisk the egg whites until stiff, then add the dietor a little at a time and finally a few drops of lemon, so you have made your own ice that you will need to decorate.

The biscuits are served cold and you can decorate them as you like, with the help of a pastry bag filled with your ice cream.

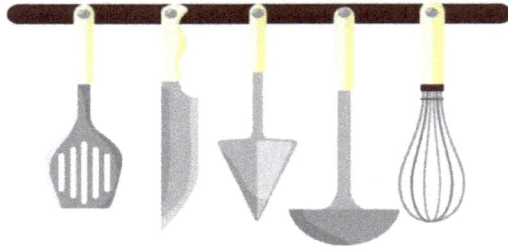

JAM OF BANANAS

GLUTEN FREE

Times:

Preparation 15 min

Cooking 5/6 min

Bain-marie 45 min

Total 65/66 min

For 4 jars of 250 grams

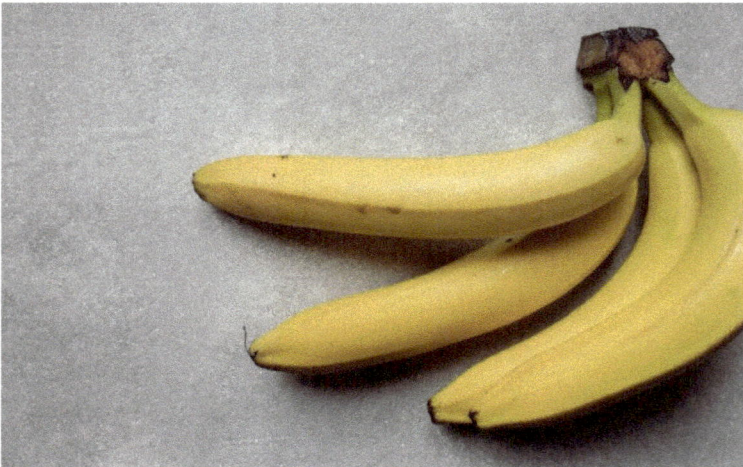

For 1 jar:

Nutritional values

Calories 210

Carbohydrates 1.27 gr

Ratio 2.46 gr

Fats 19.09 gr

Protein 6.49 gr

MATERIALS

1 Terrine

1 Hand blender

4 glass jars of about 250 gr with cap

1 saucepan

INGREDIENTS

800 gr of ripe bananas net

juice of one lemon

400 grams of fine brown sugar

q. b. vanilla or cinnamon powder (optional)

INSTRUCTIONS

To prepare the jam, start by peeling the bananas, cut the pulp into small pieces, finally put it in a bowl, now add the lemon juice, in this way the banana pulp will not become dark, put the bananas in the pot, add the zest of lemon, brown sugar and mix well, now you can add a little cinnamon or vanilla powder to give it the aroma, more or less one or the other according to your tastes.

Cook for about 5/6 minutes over medium / low heat, then blend the bananas using an immersion blender, continue to blend until the mixture is fluffy and homogeneous.

Pour the confettura in jars, turn them upside down and wait for them to cool.

Put them in a water bath for about 45 minutes, to remove the air so that they can be kept under vacuum for a long time. Keep the jam in a cool and dry place for three weeks before using it, to fill pancakes or to spread it on bread or to eat it alone for breakfast.

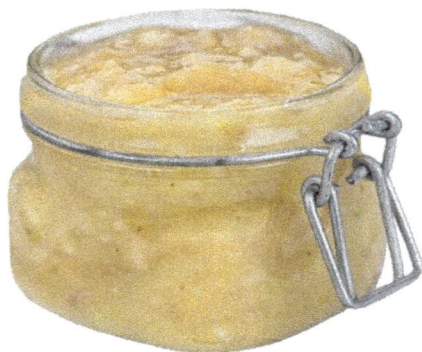

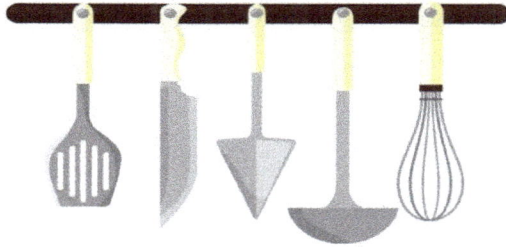

CROISSANT / CORNETTI

Puff pastry is a basic element of the kitchen, which can be used for wonderful sweet and savory preparations. For this classic gluten-free croissant we decided to start from the dough and the folding of the puff pastry itself, without fear of the complexity of the folds and processing in general. As is known, puff pastry requires several steps. The dough is folded several times and spread on itself, gradually adding layers of butter or margarine. A fragrant croissant in the oven smells good, instilling joy for the whole house. Treat yourself to this pampering and the day will flow lightly and always with a beautiful smile.

GLUTEN FREE

Times:

Preparation 25 min

Rising 2 hours

Cooking 30 min

Total 2 hours and 55 min

For 10 croissants

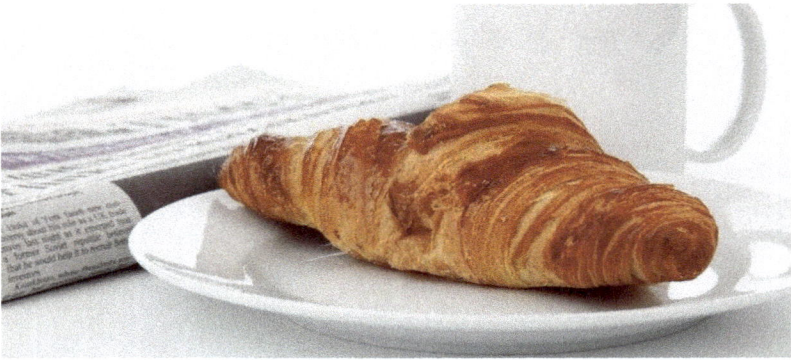

For 1 croissant:

Nutritional values

Calories 171

Carbohydrates 24 gr

Sugars 4 gr

Fats 5 gr

Protein 10 gr

MATERIALS

Puff pastry or rolling pin machine

Mixer or planetary

1 baking sheet

Greaseproof paper

INGREDIENTS

500 gr of sweet gold puff pastry mix

260 grams of water

30 grams of sunflower oil

35 gr of fresh yeast

Zest 1 grated lemon

Zest of 1 grated orange

2 bourbon vanilla pods

270 gr of vegetable margarine

INSTRUCTIONS

Put the sweet gold puff pastry mix in the bowl of the planetary mixer and mix well for a couple of minutes at medium speed, put the yeast in warm water and dissolve it, continue to knead the mixture, pouring the yeast and adding the oil and the aromas, until to form a loaf, soft and homogeneous. Take the dough and roll it out with a rolling pin or, better still, with the dough sheeter, the puff pastry machine, roll out the dough until it reaches a thickness of about 7 millimeters.

On a sheet of baking paper, cut out the margarine and cover it with another sheet of paper. Roll out the margarine to a thickness of 12 millimeters and lay it on the sheet of the previously spread dough, folding to form 3 folds of 3, in 3 steps. At the end of the folds you will have to obtain a dough with a thickness of about 7 millimeters. Then proceed to cut out the triangles that will serve as a base for the croissants. Each triangle must have dimensions of 3 × 1 cm. Before rolling the triangle on itself, moisten the surface with a brush wet with water. After having composed all the croissants in this way, put them to rise on a baking sheet lined with parchment paper and leave them at a stable temperature of 30 ° degrees for 2 hours.

Once the leavening is complete, heat the oven to 175 ° degrees
and finish with cooking for 30 minutes.

Let it cool and serve.

Enjoy your meal!

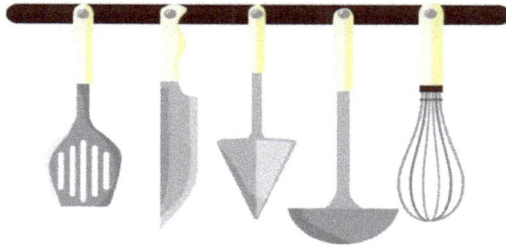

TARTS OF ORANGE JAM

Milk makes the difference in this recipe for tartlets with orange jam, it must be strictly lactose-free.

Much lighter and more digestible, it is ideal for the intolerant, but also for all those who do not suffer from intolerances.

GLUTEN FREE

LACTOSE-FREE

Times:

Preparation 20 min

Cooking 30 min

Total 50 min

For 8 tarts

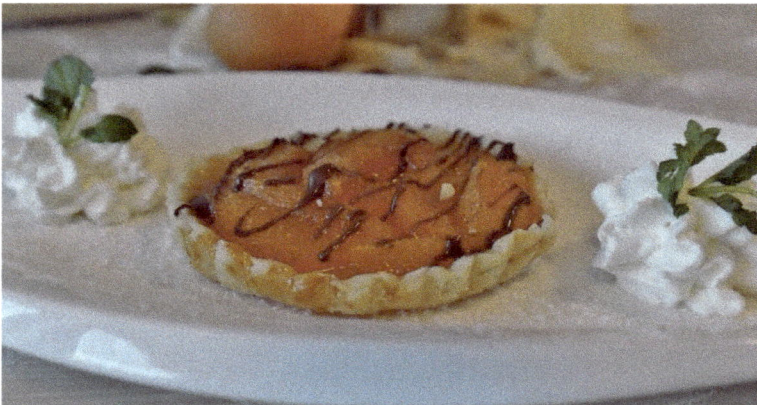

For 1 tart:

Nutritional values

Calories 245

Net carbohydrates 6 gr

Fat 19 gr

Protein 10 gr

MATERIALS

2 Bowls

1 small saucepan

Greaseproof paper

10 baking molds with a diameter

of about 8/10 cm

INGREDIENTS

200 gr of sorghum flour

100 gr of brown rice flour

80 grams of whole cane sugar

50 gr of potato starch

80 ml of rice oil

80 ml of water

2 teaspoons of gluten-free baking powder

grated zest of organic orange or lemon

2 tablespoons of lactose-free milk

q.s. of orange marmalade without sugar

INSTRUCTIONS

Start this recipe, put the 2 types of flours in a bowl, after sifting them, add the starch, the baking powder and the grated rind of the lemon or orange to your liking and then mix all the ingredients well.

In another bowl, dissolve the sugar in the water, then pour the rice oil, the milk, mix all the ingredients well and then add the flour.

Work the mixture well with your hands, until you get a soft and elastic dough.

Take molds with a diameter of about 8/10 cm, butter and flour them well, or put some parchment paper, put a little pastry to cover the surface and prick the bottom with a fork, then stuff with a generous layer of orange marmalade, level the surface of the jam with a spoon and decorate with smears short crust pastry line forming grids.

Bake the tarts in a preheated oven at 180 degrees, preferably ventilated, for about 25/30 minutes, until they are golden and cooked.

Let them cool completely and they will be ready to eat.

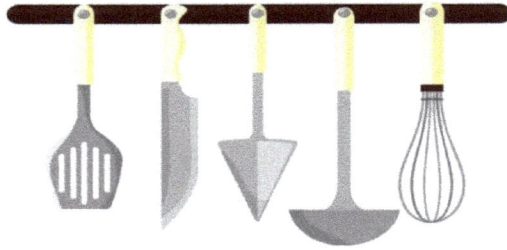

VALENTINE'S DAY CAKE WITH PISTACHIO

This is a recipe for making a cake for a special day.
The heart-shaped Valentine's Day cake with cheese and
pistachios will be perfect at the end of an accurate dinner,
obviously respecting the ketogenic,
gluten-free and lactose-free diet.

GLUTEN FREE

LACTOSE-FREE

Times:

Preparation 35 min

Cooking 15 min

Total 50 min

For 6 people

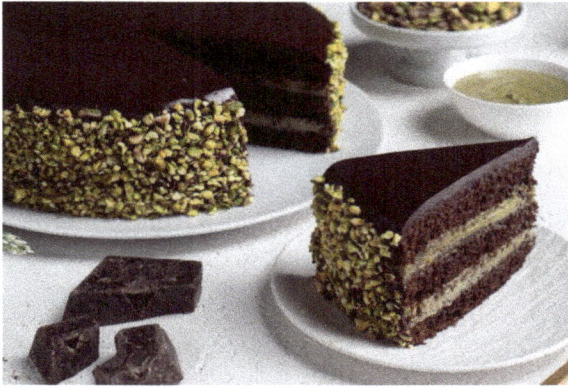

For 1 person:

Nutritional values

Calories 250

Carbohydrates 3 gr

Sugars 4 gr

Fats 18.5 gr

Protein 13.5 gr

MATERIALS

Electric whips

1 bowl

1 sieve

1 Heart-shaped mold

1 small saucepan

Coppapasta or molds

of your choice for decoration

INGREDIENTS

For the sponge cake

250 grams of whole eggs

100 grams of brown sugar

50 grams of agave syrup

150 grams of fonio flour

50 grams of pea flour

For the wet

100 g of water

50 gr agave syrup

q. b. of vanilla

For the filling and decoration

300 grams of cream

300 gr of Exquisa classic spreadable cheese

60 gr of blended pistachios and reduced to paste

30 gr of toasted pistachios in grains

q.s. sugar paste

INSTRUCTIONS

Break the eggs and put them in a large bowl and whisk them with the electric whisk together with the brown sugar and the agave syrup, until you get a very frothy and homogeneous mixture, at this point add the sifted flours a little at a time, always continuing to mount.

Take a heart-shaped mold, grease it or oil it and flour it carefully, then pour the mixture inside and bake it at 180 degrees in a preheated oven for about 10/15 minutes. Meanwhile the base is cooking in the oven, take a saucepan and start preparing the syrup *, bring the water to a boil with the agave syrup and vanilla, after boiling turn off the heat and let it cool.

So take the Exquisa spreadable cheese and add it to the pistachio paste, whipping everything with an electric whisk. Once you have finished mixing all the ingredients and left the sponge cake to cool, dedicate yourself to assembling the cake. Cut the sponge cake in half, horizontally. Wet the base disc of sponge cake with the syrup / wet previously prepared and sprinkle with the chopped pistachios, lay the second disc of sponge cake and wet it further.

Put everything in the fridge for a few hours to rest, take the sponge cake and cover it with a layer of Exquisa cheese and pistachio filling, taking care to cover the entire surface of the cake.

Roll out the sugar paste to a thickness of 3 mm and cover the surface, making the sugar paste adhere well to the shape of the cake. Decorate the surface with sugar paste, cut with a pastry cutter, with other hearts or as you prefer.

Once the decoration is finished, the Valentine's cake is ready to be served.

Enjoy your meal and happy Valentine's Day!

* Wet/Bagna:

it is a very simple but essential preparation in Italian pastry, it is a syrup based on water and sugar / sweetener enriched with liqueur or with aromas or citrus peel, for this it will be an alcoholic or non-alcoholic syrup.

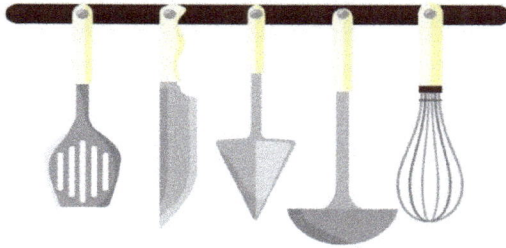

CHOCOLATE CARNIVAL PUDDING

This recipe is a little more articulated than the others, but super greedy, it was created to be made in Carnival, because it is colorful and cheerful in the presentation exactly like Carnival. By changing the decoration as you like, you can make this recipe at any time of the year, whenever you feel like eating a pudding that is healthy and good at the same time.

GLUTEN FREE

LACTOSE-FREE

Times:

Preparation 20 min

Cooling 4 hours

Total 4 hours 20 min

For 6 people

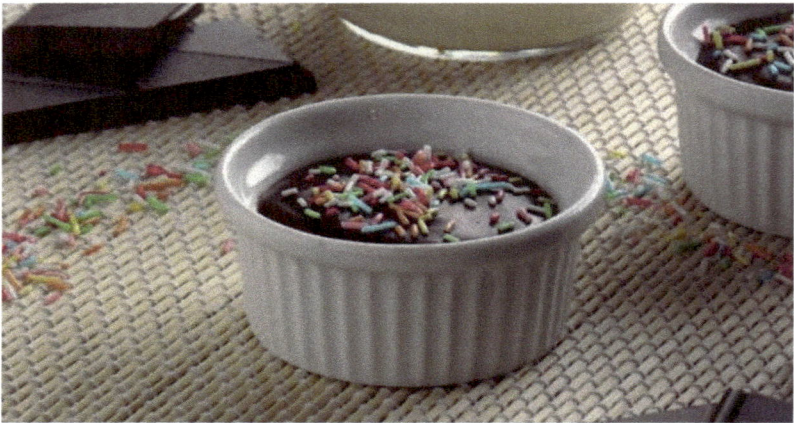

For 1 person:

Nutritional values

Calories 350

Protein 3.1 gr

Carbohydrates 11.8 gr

Fiber 1 gr

Fats 3.1 gr

MATERIALS

1 Pudding mold

1 sieve

2 pots

1 Hand whisk

INGREDIENTS

1 liter of whole milk 120 g of granulated sugar

1 teaspoon of vanillin

90 g of corn starch

70 gr of clarified butter

150 gr of 72% dark chocolate

q. b. of smarties,

sugars and colored sprinkles

INSTRUCTIONS

To prepare the chocolate pudding, start by taking the butter from the fridge and making it soften, the clarified butter will take a little longer to soften than standard butter, sift the starch well and chop the chocolate by cutting it with a knife. Now take a saucepan and put the chocolate, ghee and sugar on low heat and melt everything, mix do often with a hand whisk, in a second pan heat the milk together with a tablespoon of vanilla extract. As soon as the mixture starts to boil, add the cornstarch and mix well and carefully, making sure that no lumps form, now pour this second mixture into the first mixture that contains the chocolate and mix vigorously with a hand whisk . Then turn on the heat again and bring everything to a boil, without stopping stirring, cook over moderate heat for 5 minutes. Moisten a pudding mold with a little water and pour the mixture into it, let it cool and keep in the fridge for 4 hours. Finally, remove the pudding from the mold by turning it upside down on a large flat plate and now have fun in the decoration, garnish with smarties, sugars and colored sugared almonds.

The pudding is served!

Thanks for choosing us!

www.ingramcontent.com/pod-product-compliance
Lightning Source LLC
Chambersburg PA
CBHW041214030426
42336CB00023B/3337